I0782775

Feel, Deal, Reveal: The Teen's Journey to Emotional Freedom

Exploring and Transforming Your Inner World through Games, Mindfulness and Self-Discovery

By

Jordan Phoenix

© Copyright 2024 by Jordan Phoenix - All rights reserved.

This document is geared towards providing exact and reliable information regarding the topic and issue covered. The publication is sold with the idea that the publisher is not required to render accounting, officially permitted, or otherwise qualified services. If advice is necessary, legal, or professional, a practiced professional individual should be ordered.

From a Declaration of Principles accepted and approved equally by a Committee of the American Bar Association and a Committee of Publishers and Associations.

In no way is it legal to reproduce, duplicate, or transmit any part of this document in either electronic means or printed format. Recording this publication is strictly prohibited, and any storage of this document is not allowed unless with written permission from the publisher. All rights reserved.

The information provided herein is stated to be truthful and consistent, in that any liability, in terms of inattention or otherwise, by any usage or abuse of any policies, processes, or Instructions contained within is the solitary and utter responsibility of the recipient reader. Under no circumstances will any legal obligation or blame be held against the publisher for reparation, damages, or monetary loss due to the information herein, either directly or indirectly.

Respective authors own all copyrights not held by the publisher.

The information herein is solely offered for informational purposes and is universal. The presentation of the data is without a contract or any guaranteed assurance.

The trademarks used are without any consent, and the publication of the trademark is without permission or backing by the trademark owner. All trademarks and brands within this book are for clarifying purposes only and are owned by the owners themselves, not affiliated with this document.

Sommario

Introduction

As a parent, one might lose sight of the difficulties and changes that have occurred. It all feels like a haze that happened much too fast. The truth is that the teenage years, which go from 13 to 19, maybe the most difficult time for any developing child to deal with and navigate, particularly in today's times. Being a teenager in the digital era is undoubtedly more difficult! Hormonal and Physical changes, crucial choices to make, new experiences on the horizon, and, of course, an overflow of media make things neither easier nor better. Teenage difficulties might include bad body image, lack of self-confidence, peer pressure, low motivation, lack of attention, internet addiction, academic stress, frequent mood swings, and the list goes on. For parents, it might be a different nightmare, particularly if there is a communication breakdown between the adolescent and you.

However, not knowing what your kid is doing is scarier than knowing what they're up to. So, here's a way that may help you better understand your teenager and will undoubtedly assist him or her in coping with life's ups and downs. Pre-teen and adolescent years are ideal times to instill healthy habits in your kid. In this book, you will learn about teenagers' emotions, guiding them toward the elusive world of emoti onal liberation.

Through insightful insights, the book becomes a reliable companion, offering practical skills and activities to help develop resilience   and emotional intelligence. When we feel and emote, we release energy. This energy is not visible (at least not to all of us), but it may be felt. That is why we are attracted to some people while being repulsed by or distrustful of others. This energy, mostly released via our chakras, creates a delicate, energetic environment all around us. You may have heard of the aura. The same thing! Some individuals have a powerful, magnetic aura or field, others have a weak, fearful one, while yet others emit energy that is pleasant, compassionate, or secure. It all relies on how the individual appears, emotes, feels, talks, and behaves. Anger, despair, guilt, anxiety, and fear are more powerful emotions than joy, calm, and motivation. Negative emotions cause blockages in the energy field or energy body. Because this energy circulates across the field via passageways or meridians, any obstruction creates an impediment or traffic jam in the normal flow of energy! If these energy obstacles are not addressed or released promptly, they may accumulate and appear physically as health problems, diseases, and diseases. From overcoming self-limiting ideas to building meaningful relationships, the tips taught in this book apply to the obstacles that teenagers confront. Ultimately, this book will help youngsters towards emotional emancipation and self-acceptance, creating a generation ready to face life's complexity with increased confidence and emotional independence.

Chapter 1

Understanding Emotions

How are you feeling right now as you begin to read this? Are you curious? Hopefully, you'll discover something about yourself. Are you bored because this is a school assignment that you don't love, or are you joyful because it is a school project you adore? Perhaps you're distracted by something else, such as excitement for your weekend plans or sadness over a recent split. These kinds of emotions are natural to humans. They provide us with information about our situation and advise us on how to respond. In this chapter, you will discover everything about various emotions. So, keep on reading.

1.1 Different Emotions Teens Experience

We can detect our emotions from the time we are newborns. Infants and young children show their emotions via facial expressions or physical movements such as laughing, snuggling, or crying. They experience and express emotions, but they cannot describe them or explain why they feel the way they do. We improve our ability to comprehend emotions as we become older. Instead of responding as children do, we can recognize and express our emotions. With time and effort, we become more aware of what we are experiencing and why. This ability is known as emotional awareness. It enables us to form better connections. This is because being aware of our emotions allows us to express ourselves more clearly, avoid or settle disputes more effectively, and move beyond painful feelings more readily. Some individuals are inherently more in tune with their emotions than others.

The good news is that everyone can become more conscious of their emotions. It requires only practice. But the work is worthwhile: Emotional awareness is the first step towards developing emotional intelligence, a talent that may help individuals thrive in their lives.

Here are some fundamental facts regarding emotions:

- Emotions come and go. Most of us experience a variety of emotions during the day. Some endure just a few seconds. Others may develop into a mood.

- Emotions may range from mild to severe. The strength of an emotion varies depending on the environment and the individual.

- Emotions are not inherently good or evil, yet there are appropriate and inappropriate methods to express them. Learning how to express emotions in appropriate ways is a different skill called emotion management, which is based on the foundation of understanding emotions.

Some emotions feel positive, such as happiness, confidence, love, inspiration, cheerfulness, gratitude, interest, or inclusion. Other emotions might seem more negative, such as anger, fear, resentment, humiliation, sadness, guilt, or worry. It is common to have both happy and negative feelings. Every emotion reveals something about us and our circumstances. However, we occasionally struggle to embrace our feelings. We may condemn ourselves for experiencing certain emotions, such as jealousy. Instead of telling ourselves that we shouldn't feel that way, we should pay attention to how we truly feel.

Avoiding bad sensations or claiming we don't experience them might have the opposite effect. It is more difficult to go beyond uncomfortable sentiments and let them go if we do not confront them and attempt to understand why we feel the way we do. You do not need to focus on your feelings or continuously express how you feel. Emotional awareness is just recognizing, appreciating, and accepting your emotions as they occur. Emotions, like everything else in life, need practice to master! Remind yourself that there are no positive or negative feelings. Don't criticize your emotions; instead, keep observing and identifying them.

Emotional Ups and Downs: A Teen's Experience

- **Physical factors**

   Adolescence brings about several bodily changes for pre-teens and adolescents. Your child's body is changing, which may make them feel self-conscious or ashamed - or just desire more solitude and time alone. Pre-teens and adolescents who seem to grow sooner or later than their peers may have emotional responses to these physical changes.

   Another physical element is sleep. Pre-teens need 9 to 11 hours of sleep, whereas adolescents need 8-10 hours. The quantity of sleep your kid receives is likely to influence their mood. Your child's dietary and nutritional habits, as well as their degree of physical activity, may all have an impact on their mood. A healthy diet and regular exercise may frequently help your kid control his or her mood.

- **Brain factors**

  The adolescent brain undergoes several changes throughout the teen years. For example, brain changes stimulate your child's body to produce sex hormones. These hormones cause bodily changes, as well as romantic and sexual emotions. These new emotions might be intense and perplexing for your youngster. Also, your child's brain will continue to change into their early twenties. The prefrontal cortex, the final portion of the brain to mature is intimately related to the areas involved in emotional regulation and management. This implies that your kid may struggle to regulate some of their stronger emotions, and they may seem to respond more intensely to circumstances than before. They're still figuring out how to analyze and express their feelings as adults.

- **Social and emotional variables.**

  New ideas, feelings, friends, and responsibilities may all influence how your kid feels. Your youngster is learning to solve more difficulties on their own as they progress towards independence. Your youngster is also more reflective than usual, preoccupied with issues such as friendships, school, and family ties. Stressful family conditions might also affect your child's mood.

How to Help teenagers and pre-teens manage their emotional ups and downs

You cannot prevent your youngster from feeling flat or low. However, there are several things you can do to assist your kid cope with the ups and downs.

- **Helping your youngster accept the ups and downs.**

  It may assist your youngster in understanding that emotional fluctuations are normal parts of life. One of the most effective ways to do this is to communicate to your kid that you, too, have moments of flatness. It's also crucial for your kid to know that you'll be there for them when they're down or going through a difficult moment. You do not need to fix your child's difficulties. Instead, just saying, 'I see you're having a rough day' might be helpful. This reassures your youngster that it is normal to feel low or flat at times.

- **Staying close to your kid**

  Staying engaged and actively listening to what's going on in your child's life can allow you to more readily identify the triggers because of their emotional ups and downs. Casual, ordinary activities, such as driving your kid someplace or watching TV together, may be excellent opportunities for your youngster to share with you.

- **Giving your kid space**

  Your youngster is gaining independence and trying new things. While this is occurring, try to allow your kid some alone time to process new feelings and experiences. Let your youngster know you'll be available if they want to chat.

- **Holding off on solutions.**

If there is a problem, brainstorming solutions with your kid might be beneficial, but your youngster must participate in the solutions and believe that they 'own' them. Your youngster is more likely to attempt the remedy if they believe it came from them.

Also, problem-solving is an important life skill that your kid will improve with practice. Helping your kid develop problem-solving abilities sends the message that you appreciate their involvement in life-changing choices.

- **Working together on coping techniques.**

One of the most important aspects of adolescence is learning to deal with and handle emotional ups and downs on one's own. You may also assist your youngster in learning this vital life skill.

One method to do this is to create a list of ' mood busters' with your youngster. These are activities that your youngster can undertake to feel better. Consider listening to energetic or beloved music.

- Spend time with a buddy.

- Take a quick stroll.

- Pat a dog.

- Receive a hug from you.

- Enjoy a movie with you.

It is beneficial for your kid to have a variety of alternatives on their list so that they may experiment and find what works best.

- **Becoming a role model**

You are still your child's most significant role model. Your youngster will turn to you to see how you handle difficult circumstances. Consider how your youngster perceives your problem-solving abilities and coping skills.

Feeling sad or flat regularly might sometimes indicate a more severe issue.

Pre-teens and young people may experience feelings of depression lasting minutes, hours, days, or even weeks. If your kid seems depressed, angry, flat, or unhappy for more than two weeks, or if mood swings prevent your child from engaging in their typical daily activities, this might be an indication of a more severe mental health issue.

If you are worried about your child's feelings and conduct, you should speak with them and get support from a mental health specialist. Your general practitioner may assist you in finding the appropriate individual. Most pre-teens and adolescents with mental health issues recover well with therapy, especially if they get it early.

1.2 Tools and Techniques to Recognize Emotions

Do you ever have sensations that you can't identify? Perhaps you're feeling more teary than normal, and the simplest thing triggers you. Perhaps there is a seething fury that you don't understand. While emotional literacy is typically given more attention in elementary school, by the time children get to middle and high school, they are "figuring out who they are and how they want to stand up in the world." During these crucial and transitional years, kids need skills to understand and manage their complicated emotions due to their developing brains and the psychological fluctuations that accompany puberty.

This list comprises techniques that are simple practices that a teen may use daily to process their emotions and enhance their general well-being. My main advice is that you attempt at least one of these techniques today rather than just reading about them.

So, how can we connect with our emotions? Here are some options to try. Let's get started.

- **Write it out.**

    This is my private go-to, as someone who has maintained a notebook since the age of thirteen. Writing down how you feel might help you organize your ideas and emotions and put them on paper. The act of putting pen to paper is therapeutic for many.

- **Feel it in your own body.**

Our emotions may manifest physically, particularly when we are unable to recognize or comprehend them. This is something that somatic therapy may assist with. The method employs physical exercises and techniques to help you stay present in your body and connect with your emotions. Somatic therapy may assist with a variety of issues, such as trauma, anxiety, chronic pain, and depression.

- **Get inventive.**

Taking a more conceptual approach to emotions might sometimes provide the distance we need to connect with them. This is the concept of many arts treatments, which may be quite helpful. Here are a few innovative ideas:

- Paint a landscape of your feelings.

- Write a short tale about a character who shares your feelings.

- Create a playlist to express your emotions.

- Don't worry if what comes out doesn't make sense at first; keep writing and consider what drew you to certain colors, narrative ideas, or tunes. Allow yourself to softly explore.

- **Watch an emotional movie or TV program.**

When I know I have grief in my chest but can't let it out, I watch a TV program. This frequently helps to relieve my melancholy by allowing me to weep, not just for the people on television but also for myself. Sometimes, a plot strikes a deeper chord than others, and we may wonder why we should explore our feelings.

- **Name it to tame it.**

When we are emotionally overloaded, it seems as if we are in a fog. We can't put our finger on how we feel; all we know is that something is wrong, and we feel terrible. Our emotions might leave us feeling confused and uncomfortable, leading us to seek distractions such as chocolate, email, or kitten videos.

First and foremost, I want you to understand that doesn't feel good is very normal. We all feel this way at times. We may admit our bad, complicated emotional condition and strive to move one step further. And it is 'Name your emotion'. There are four basic emotions: sad, furious, pleased, and afraid. This basic schema is likely a nice place to begin.

Our emotional intelligence relies heavily on expanding our emotional lexicon. Verbalization allows us to comprehend and express ourselves. Once we understand the feeling we are dealing with, we can extract what we need from it and go on.

- **Dance to it**

An emotion is a kind of energy in motion. To digest it, we must express it. We need to relocate. The problem is that many of us do not have a secure place to feel and express our feelings. We can learn a lot from youngsters who stamp their feet, shout, clench their fists, or fall on the floor and weep in despair, even if they are in the midst of a supermarket. We can and should make room for ourselves to express our feelings in absolutely stupid ways when no one is looking. Do you know what may serve as a trigger for this practice? Music.

- Choose a few songs and dance to convey your deepest feelings.

- To express rage, use physical actions such as stomping, punching, or yelling into a pillow.

- For anxiousness, try shaking, running, or jumping up and down.

- To relieve grief, roll on the floor, move gently, relax your muscles, and collapse.

Express your feelings or an emotion you have previously ignored in a secure atmosphere, away from everyone's gaze. It may seem not very intelligent at first, but it will feel therapeutic and energizing after you're finished. This should be a practice, so choose many songs and create several choreographies for your typical feelings.

- **Breathe through it**

Our breath may work wonders for our health, vitality, and, yes, emotions. It has regained appeal thanks to meditation, yoga, and the recent work of James Nestor and other pulmonologist (those who harness the power of breathing). Many transformational breathing methods, including box breathing, alternate nostril breathing, and 4-7-8 breathing, may help you relax and reduce anxiety.

However, one method is pranayama breathing meditation or two-part active breathwork. This method includes mouth breathing in a specific pattern:

- Inhale deeply into your abdomen.

- Inhale deeply into your chest.

- Exhale via your mouth.

This rhythm is performed for a certain amount of time (ten minutes to an hour), usually accompanied by music. An equal amount of rest follows the interval of vigorous breathing. What occurs in the process is nothing short of amazing. You will feel the energy flowing through your body. You may experience tingles in the hands, face, and legs, a decrease in your body temperature, intense emotional surges, shaking, tears, yelling, visions, new thoughts, and a total change in your energy. The effects and advantages of this treatment are comparable to those of acupuncture.

Breathwork is powerful, so start with shorter sessions and practice with the facilitator. With time, you'll be able to accomplish it on your own, requiring just a music playlist and a quiet location. Because it is so visceral and powerful, this exercise is straightforward and convenient, requiring little attention. Consider it mental hygiene: brushing the dust off your emotional body, washing and restoring.

- **Emotional Freedom Technique (EFT)**

EFT, commonly known as tapping, involves tapping on several energy points on the body and face. You'll be talking about the emotions (or whatever else is the topic of your tapping session) while processing them both logically and viscerally. What you can enjoy about EFT, in particular, is that it incorporates strong messages of self-love, compassion, and acceptance, as well as the ability to gently adjust our viewpoint while being aware of where we are.

1.3 Understanding the Neuroscience of Emotions

The brain is the neediest organ in your body. It takes more nutrients and oxygen rather than any other, and the intricate brain networks that comprise it account for the majority of what you perform each day. Neuroscience advances have increased our knowledge of complicated emotions and actions, offering useful information for our everyday lives. When asked what makes you human, emotions - or some component of your personality that is inextricably tied to emotions - may rank near the top of the list. Our emotions have an impact on our relationships, lifestyle, career, sense of self, and choices, both large and small. Darwin was also captivated by emotions and thought that emotions exist to alert us immediately if a situation is safe. In these and many other ways, we understand the value of our emotions. We understand that fear helps us cross the road safely, anger gives us power, and love keeps us connected to others. We could repress and dismiss the ones we don't want or don't think are 'proper' while pursuing the ones we want, perhaps to our cost.

Our brain is covered with neural networks, which get weaker or stronger depending on how often they are utilized. Repeated usage creates incredibly powerful 'neural highways', which establish our default thinking, personality, and emotional profile. The good news is that we can remodel our brain pathways via a process known as neuroplasticity. So, what are the primary emotions at the core of our brain networks? The human emotion spectrum consists of eight primary emotions: sorrow, humiliation, anger, disgust, fear, excitement/joy, startle/surprise, and love/trust. As you may have observed, we are all a bit imbalanced, with more main emotions accessible to us on the side of the scale that represents 'escape' rather than 'attachment'. Unfortunately, evolutionarily speaking, it was more vital for us to be safe than to have fun.

- Sadness indicates a problem in our situation.

- Shame serves as a moral compass, but it may be damaging if overemphasized in certain circumstances. Our response to shame may either force us to retreat from the activity that resulted in this sensation or motivate us to try harder to prevent the feeling the next time around.

- Disgust evolved to protect humans from microbial damage. Disgust prevents us from eating spoiled food and keeps us away from other things that we believe are harmful to our health.

- Anger attempts to alter the circumstance. It's not passive, like melancholy. Anger's usefulness varies depending on the scenario. Fear arises when we recognize a threat and feel helpless to prevent it. Fear stimulates the fight or flight reaction.

- Surprises may be both positive and negative. When we are surprised, we have no idea what will happen, so our brain and body use additional energy to prepare for what may occur. Endorphins flood the brain, making us feel calmer.

- Excitement and delight are motivated by pleasure and reward.

- Love and trust are based on predictability. These feelings accumulate as we create a backlog of pleasant, reinforcing events and memories involving another person. These emotions also take into consideration how individuals, including this new person, have treated you in the past.

Parts of the brain involved in the Emotional response

Many major regions contribute to how emotions operate in the brain. The prefrontal cortex, which occurs in the human brain, is responsible for emotional management and decision-making. This is where we keep our sense of ourselves, our value system, and our willpower. We utilize the prefrontal cortex to repress emotions. The next important region is the amygdala. Our amygdala scans our surroundings for possible danger and generates the fear, anxiety, and rage that we may need to react to that risk. The amygdala is also where we keep emotional memories. Our thalamus collects information from the senses (sight, smell, touch, hearing, and taste) and transfers it to the appropriate parts of the brain. The hippocampus is where we store memories. We also utilize it to navigate. The hippocampus preserves bodily feelings of emotion.

How do these regions interact during an anxious response?

While our amygdala has been extremely beneficial to our survival throughout evolution, people suffering from anxiety disorders may have an overactive amygdala that views danger and threat disproportionately, flooding the brain and the body with the same emotions that we may have needed in the past to avoid real predatory dangers. When we see something that causes us to experience dread or worry, our thalamus transmits this information to the amygdala. The amygdala communicates with our brain to determine if we have any memories that might help us understand how to respond in the current scenario. If our hippocampus recalls traumatic emotional memories, we experience dread and anxiety. Strong emotions might lead the logical brain to shut down. Our amygdala is faster at responding than our reasoning brain. Anxiety and dread cause shallow breathing, which deprives the brain of oxygen and forces regions of the brain that are not engaged in survival to take a back seat. We are unable to think rationally, creatively, or with empathy. Breathing exercises may, therefore, be quite beneficial while feeling dread or anxiety; ensuring that the brain receives the oxygen it needs to operate correctly can help you better manage your emotions.

Feelings, Emotions, and moods

Typically, we feel emotions in reaction to a particular external input, although this is not always the case. Our ideas may also cause emotional reactions. If our human brain recalls a memory or concept of a period when we felt shame or rage, the mammal brain may be prompted to produce a bodily emotional response. These are emotions. Feelings, unlike emotions, may be rationalized. An emotion occurs rapidly; emotions are reactions to our surroundings paired with our interpretations, ideas, or inner beliefs about the circumstance. As a result, our feelings are more controllable than our emotions: we can examine our sentiments, mirror our ideas back to ourselves, and challenge their validity. Moods and Emotions are also unique. Emotions are quick, distinct reactions to particular events that tell us about our present circumstances, although moods are far more difficult to identify. Moods generally have a more gradual start, and it is unclear what causes them. Moods provide information about our present state of being and our inner system. Unlike emotions, moods are detrimental to decision-making. Emotions are important in decision-making because they provide information about our present condition. We are often taught that there is a distinction between 'following your mind' and 'following the heart', with the latter commonly associated with being dumb or illogical. However, ignoring your emotions while making decisions may lead to chronic uncertainty. Refusing to pay attention to what your emotions are saying might put you in a stressful condition of 'paralysis and analysis', preventing you from moving ahead. We may believe that life would be simpler if our feelings were more predictable, tranquil, or just less prevalent, yet they are one of our most valuable resources and are eventually here to serve us.

1.4 Benefits of being in Tune with Your Feelings

Emotional awareness is the capacity to name one's conscious experience of affect with an emotion-related term. Emotions are physiologically grounded patterns of experience, perception, physiology, behavior, and communication that our brains produce for cultural purposes. Emotion is founded on affect, which is the bodily sense of pleasure and discomfort. We are born with affect, not with feelings.

In early life, we learn emotions by compiling a database of physical events and emotional phrases. We feel the effects bodily. When we are aware of a bodily sensation, we experience emotion. Here is one example. Suppose anything occurs to me. I am experiencing a little negative influence of anger/rage. I become aware of the feeling I'm experiencing. Using my emotional database, I can define the sense as irritation. I am aware that I am having feelings of irritation.

Advantages of Being Emotionally Aware

- **Stronger leadership qualities**

  An emotionally skilled leader can read their team's feelings. This helps a leader decide how to approach projects, inspire team members, and assess performance.

- **Reduced levels of social anxiety.**

  Emotional awareness reduces social anxiety. Research suggests a link between social anxiety and a lack of emotional control. If you suffer from social anxiety, you are unable to control your emotions. This means that socially worried persons are emotionally unaware. Increasing emotional awareness tends to reduce social anxiety.

- **Improved relationships with family and friends.**

  Relationships are built on emotions rather than reason. If you are mindful of your emotions, you will be sensitive to the sentiments of your family and friends. You will understand and connect to them more deeply than if you were emotionally detached.

- **Higher self-esteem.**

  Emotional awareness boosts confidence and self-esteem since it allows you to handle challenging emotional circumstances that the oblivious cannot. You can deal with challenging talks and uncomfortable disputes and end disagreements and battles. You can regulate your emotions.

Chapter 2

Practical Self-Regulation Strategies

Self-regulation is essential for sustaining emotional well-being, overcoming life's adversities, and completing objectives. In this chapter, you will learn some practical self-regulation strategies that you may use in your everyday life.

2.1 Simple Practices for Immediate Stress Relief

We've compiled a list of six stress-management strategies for you on this topic:

- **Maintain your physical fitness.**

  It may seem obvious, but exercising via walking, running, gardening, or any other activity that keeps you moving is one of the most effective methods to reduce stress. According to the Mayo Clinic, "virtually any form of workout can act as a stress reliever," and exercise boosts feel-good endorphins and other natural neurochemicals. Eating a variety of vegetables, fruits, and whole grains is also beneficial.

  Sunbasket, for example, provides services that promote healthier eating habits. Sunbasket, co-founded by San Francisco chef Justine Kelly, is a meal kit delivery business that provides recipes and materials for healthy, homemade meals. The firm also claims it monitors its carbon impact and strives to provide just the quantity of food required for each meal, minimizing food waste.

- **Practice meditation.**

Meditation, which focuses on calming the mind, is another popular stress-management technique. It has been practiced for numerous years, yet there are new techniques to achieve zen.

- **Keep a journal.**

There are several methods to journal that may enhance your mental health and reduce stress in your life, including daily affirmations, venting, expressing gratitude, manifesting, and more. If you're new to journaling and don't know where to start, there are several guided notebooks or mental health workbooks available.

Molly Burford, an author and social media strategist, wrote "The No Worries Workbook," which has 124 lists, exercises, and suggestions to "get out of your head and carry on with your life. It was designed to "turn toxic positivity on its head" by presenting "cathartic" ways of venting and gratitude writing, including plenty of cursing and encouragement to switch off any unpleasant ideas in your life.

- **Maintain a routine.**

Similar to blogging, keeping a timetable or planning your day out in the mornings will help you avoid hassles. Writing in a paper planner, rather than your online Google Calendar, may help you remember all you need to accomplish for the day, week, month, or year. It enables you to take a 10-minute break from your displays.

- **Try Breathing exercises**

   This relaxing breathing method for stress, anxiety, and panic requires just a few minutes and can be performed anywhere. The biggest advantage will come from doing it regularly as part of your daily routine. You may practice it standing, sitting in a back-supporting chair, or reclining on your bed or yoga mat on the floor. Make yourself as comfortable as possible. If possible, loosen any clothing that is restricting your breathing. If you're lying down, position your arms slightly away from your sides, palms up. Keep your legs straight or bend the knees so your feet are flat on the ground. If you are seated, rest your arms on the chair arms. If you're seated or standing, keep both feet flat on the floor. Place your feet about hip-width apart, regardless of your posture.

1. Take a deep, comfortable breath into your belly without straining it.

2. Try inhaling through the nose and exhaling through your mouth.

3. Inhale slowly and frequently. Some individuals find it beneficial to count consistently from one to five. You may be unable to reach 5 at first.

4. Gently let it out, counting from 1 to 5 as needed.

5. Do this for a minimum of 5 minutes.

2.2 Cognitive Restructuring for Changing Negative Thought Patterns

Cognitive restructuring strategies break down problematic ideas and reconstruct them in a more balanced and correct manner. Most individuals have negative thinking patterns from time to time, but these patterns may become so ingrained that they impair relationships, accomplishments, and even well-being.

Cognitive restructuring is a set of therapy strategies that help individuals recognize and modify harmful thought habits. When harmful and self-defeating thinking patterns emerge, mental health specialists may assist you in exploring strategies for interrupting and redirecting them.

What is the mechanism of cognitive restructuring?

Cognitive restructuring is central to cognitive behavioral therapy, a well-studied talk therapy technique that successfully treats a wide range of mental health disorders. This includes:

- anxiety disorders

- depression

- eating disorders

- personality disorders

- substance use disorders

Cognitive behavioral therapy (CBT) involves working with a behavior therapist to discover and practice skills for reshaping problematic thinking patterns. Psychologists, Psychiatrists, and other mental health experts specialize in cognitive behavioral therapy. It might be difficult to identify errors in your mental habits. As a result, specialists usually advocate working with a therapist while starting cognitive restructuring. People may have cognitive distortions, which are thinking processes that generate a mistaken perception of reality. These cognitive patterns often result in anxiety, depression, relational troubles, and self-destructive behaviors.

Some examples of cognitive distortions include:

- catastrophizing

- black-and-white thinking

- Personalization

- Overgeneralization

Cognitive restructuring allows you to detect these maladaptive beliefs as they occur. You may then practice reframing things more truthfully and helpfully. The notion holds that if you can modify your perspective on certain events or situations, you may be able to change your emotions and behaviors.

What are the benefits?

Although it is beneficial to work with a counselor at first, cognitive restructuring is a technique that can be learned on your own once you understand how it works. Being able to recognize and modify your negative thinking patterns offers several advantages. For example, it might assist to:

• Reduce stress and anxiety

• Improve communication skills and relationships

• Replace harmful coping strategies like drug use

• Boost self-confidence and self-esteem

In every circumstance where negative thinking patterns emerge, cognitive restructuring may assist you in challenging and changing harmful ideas.

Cognitive restructuring techniques

Teenagers often engage in negative self-talk by focusing their negative thoughts inward. Teenagers tend to be severe judges of themselves and believe that others feel the same way instead of being sympathetic advocates for themselves. Cognitive reframing includes the practice of talking to oneself with love and compassion. By using these Cognitive Behavioral Therapy techniques (CBT) strategies, teenagers may improve their sense of confidence and self-worth. Adolescents who use positive self-talk also teach their brains to focus on possibilities and strengths rather than defects and issues. Teens may rephrase statements like "I'm bad at X" to "I'm still learning how to do X" by using positive self-talk. Alternatively, "I messed everything up" might be rephrased as "I can do it differently the next time because I see what didn't work well."

The ABCDE approach is a cognitive restructuring strategy that involves:

A = the **A**ctivating event linked with negative thoughts

B= the **B**eliefs that may lead to negative emotions

C= the **C**onsequences related to the activating event

D = the process of **D**isputing the negative beliefs

E=Effecting one's thoughts and emotions about the stimulating event

2.3 How Teens Can Be Mindful

Being a teenager is tough! Whether it's friends, school, or dating, the teen years are filled with tough mental and physical changes. If you are like many teenagers, you may struggle to cope with stress effectively. You are not alone, and there are steps you can take to keep calm no matter how hectic life gets. All you have to do is pause, breathe, and remain alert and aware in the current moment. In this fascinating book, a pediatrician who specializes in teen and adolescent medicine presents a groundbreaking mindfulness program to help you cope with stress in healthy ways, enhance communication, and resolve disputes with family and friends. This entertaining and one-of-a-kind handbook employs mindfulness-based practices to help you stay calm under stress. The basic and easy-to-remember suggestions in this book may be utilized daily to help you cope with life's most difficult circumstances, such as taking an exam at school, dealing with your parents, or managing trouble with friends. This book will teach you how to remain cool, calm, and collected no matter what your life throws at you. If you want to discover your inner power and resilience via attentive awareness and take control of your life, this book will teach you how.

Mindfulness is the practice of paying complete attention to the present moment without judgment. Many hobbies may be done thoughtfully, including exercising, drawing, coloring, and fishing. Teens may also benefit from mindfulness exercises and methods such as timed breathing, grounding, and body scans. Mindfulness is the purposeful act of paying your full attention to the present moment (rather than the past or future) without judgment. A non-judgmental attitude is essential because we tend to criticize our ideas, and even being aware of them may result in a profound transformation. Mindfulness for children and teenagers may be an excellent method for growth and dealing with stressful situations.

Benefits of Practicing Mindfulness

Mindfulness may help individuals become more mindful of their emotions and thoughts, which can lead to new opportunities. Observing the present moment without judgment is a major aspect of mindfulness; learning to meet oneself without judgment may help one develop compassion and kindness.

Concentration is challenging in today's fast-paced media environment. Many mindfulness practices promote prolonged attention, which may help improve this ability.

Research has indicated the following advantages of mindfulness for teenagers:

- Improves optimism,

- Improves social behaviors, focus, self-control, bullying, adolescent stress, and anxiety

- Improves compassion, emotion management, and school behavior.

Mindful Practices for Teens

Mindfulness practices that meet your requirements may be practiced daily. It is OK to begin practicing mindfulness by experimenting with different strategies to find which ones work best for you. Varied hobbies may also have varied advantages; for example, some may promote relaxation while others promote alertness. Teenagers may practice mindfulness in several ways, including mental, physical, emotional, and spiritual.

Here are some mindfulness exercises for teenagers:

1. **Deep breathing.**

   Breathwork is a traditional mindfulness technique that involves actively altering the breath while attentively concentrating on it. This practice involves taking deep, slow breaths (also known as belly breaths) using the diaphragm. This prompts your muscles to relax.

2. **Paced breathing (for example inhale 5 and exhale 7).**

Paced breathing is another sort of breathwork in which the lengths of inhales and exhales are deliberately adjusted. It may be beneficial to exhale longer than inhale since our heart rate decreases somewhat during the exhale. Try breathing to 5 and exhaling to 7. Use the abilities you learned in earlier tasks (deep breathing) to take diaphragmatic breaths.

3. **Progressive Muscle Relaxation.**

Progressive muscle relaxation involves tensing and relaxing particular muscle units. For example, squeeze your shoulders up to your ears and apply as much strain as possible to your shoulders and neck. Slowly count to 3 and let go of all the stress. Repeat this with all muscle groups, particularly your hands, chest, arms, and stomach.

4. **Meditate.**

There are several styles of meditation, which often include being in one physical posture and focusing on one thing, such as your breathing, a mantra, or bodily sensations. When your mind wanders, it will nonjudgmentally return to the topic of focus. Meditation may be unpleasant at first, and it may not be suitable for all ages. If it makes you uncomfortable, try alternative mindfulness practices.

5. **Body Scan.**

   A body scan is another basic mindfulness exercise. Bring your focus to different regions of your body, potentially spending 10-30 seconds on each (for example, bottoms of feet, toes, tops of feet). Observe all bodily sensations, including warmth, coldness, tension, pressure, tingling, pain, and textures. There are several guided body scans to aid with this as well.

6. **Journaling**

   Journaling may be quite mindful, particularly when done with complete focus and no judgment. Journaling may be done as a "free write," which means you write anything that comes to mind without censoring or editing. Prompts may also be used to direct your writing towards certain themes.

7. **Movement/Exercise**

   Exercise's repeated motions may become meditative if given whole focus. When tackled with a mindfulness mindset, any physical activity may be transformed into a mindfulness activity. Take a conscious stroll and observe everything around you: noises, walking sensations, temperature, nature, and local sights.

8. **Coloring**

   Coloring is an easy way to practice mindfulness. Coloring may provide a creative and joyful element to mindfulness. To make this a mindful exercise, focus your complete attention on the coloring. When the mind wanders, carefully and nonjudgmentally redirect it back to the coloring.

9. Listen to music.

Listen to a favorite music with complete focus. You can shut your eyes and listen to everything. You should also pay attention to how the music affects your mood.

10. Mindful eating.

For a quick mindfulness exercise, try deliberately eating a piece of fruit or sweets. Begin with a clementine; observe the color and texture of the fruit; peel gently; and take note of the scent. Take a bite and gently observe how it feels to consume it.

2.4 How to Manage over-whelming Emotions

Events and conversations with others or ourselves may trigger unpleasant or overpowering emotions. Some of the most common triggers for a relapse include feelings of stress, anxiety, depression, hopelessness, or overload. It is critical to have abilities to deal with and handle excessive emotional reactions. Teens may struggle to manage overwhelming emotions since they are going through a period of tremendous psychological and emotional growth. Here are some ways that might help teenagers deal with overwhelming emotions.

1. **Observe and explain the feelings.**

   Emotions are physical, cognitive, and behavioral. These components must be observed and described to better comprehend the emotional cycle. Suppose we can recognize and explain why we feel stiff and warm when we are furious or clammy, trembling, and out of breath when we are nervous. In that case, we will be better able to adopt skills and avoid harmful behavioral reactions to unpleasant emotions.

2. **Reframe any negative or overpowering ideas.**

   Coping with strong emotions relies heavily on one's thoughts. Following a triggering occurrence, we have distinct perceptions of the happenings. Emotions are self-perpetuating, and using alternate thinking when we are overwhelmed might help us stop the pattern of feeling annoyed, angry, and despairing. If we do not receive the job we want, it is easy to fall into self-defeating thinking patterns that induce pessimism and disheartenment. Instead, focus on the various chances and experiences you got throughout the interview process, as well as what you can do differently. Alternative viewpoints may also assist in alleviating unpleasant emotional responses.

3. **Become conscious of your susceptibility to unpleasant emotions.**

The popular abbreviation is HALT. Are you hungry? Are you angry? Are you lonely? Are you tired? This is vital to remember to reduce stress and the likelihood of impulsive behavior. Another vulnerability occurs when we are under the influence of alcohol or drugs. If you are conscious of your weaknesses, you may be at peace knowing that it seems worse now than it would if you had slept well, were sober, or had eaten a satisfying meal. To avoid more emotional distress, we must acknowledge our weaknesses and practice self-care.

4. **Distract.**

Distraction may be highly effective in accepting our sentiments in the present so that we do not act on them in ways that might damage us later. ACCEPTS is a handy acronym. Are there any hobbies you might try? This may be seeing a friend or treating yourself to a good supper. You may help someone by providing service and giving back. Compare your circumstances to that of another person and feel more appreciative of your own. You might attempt doing contrary to the emotion you're experiencing. If you're feeling depressed or down, listen to optimistic or inspiring music. You might also attempt to push bad feelings or ideas away. This should be a last resort for dealing with bad feelings. Finally, try self-soothing with a bubble bath, a massage, or your favorite candle.

Chapter 3

Building Self-Esteem and Confidence

The timing of self-esteem activities for teenagers will vary based on each individual's requirements. However, certain broad criteria may be considered.

Self-esteem activities might be good in early adolescence when teenagers are going through physical and emotional changes. These exercises allow youngsters to discover their abilities, create a good self-image, and better understand themselves.

3.1 Exercises to Explore and Affirm Personal Value

When kids reach middle adolescence and face new problems, self-esteem activities may help them cope with stress, build resilience, and create a feeling of self-worth. Late adolescence is a vital period when teenagers consider their future and create objectives. During this period, self-esteem exercises may help kids develop self-efficacy, set specific goals, and maintain a positive attitude toward their talents. Self-esteem changes with time. Thus, it is necessary to participate in self-esteem activities regularly, regardless of age. It is also critical to tailor the activities to each teen's interests and preferences, ensuring that they find significance and satisfaction in the process. Encourage positive self-talk to confront negative beliefs, practice gratitude journaling to concentrate on the positives, and engage in affirmations to strengthen self-belief. Teens who participate in these activities may boost their self-esteem and build a more positive self-image. Listed below are some self-esteem activities for teens:

1. **Encouragement letter to self.**

   An encouraging letter to oneself is a passionate statement that expresses unshakable support and confidence in one's skills and capabilities. This self-directed letter is an effective tool for uplifting and motivating people, especially when they are down or discouraged.

2. **Gratitude journaling.**

   Recording what one is thankful for regularly might help one make sense of all that is going on in their life. This practice may be as simple as writing down three things to be thankful for every day before sleep.

3. **Vision Board**

   A vision board is a personalized collage of pictures, statements, and affirmations representing your goals and desires. Vision boards are powerful tools for improving attention and motivation and manifesting your greatest dreams.

4. **Meditating.**

   Meditation offers youngsters different ways to boost their self-esteem. It fosters self-awareness by assisting people in understanding their ideas and feelings, which leads to self-acceptance.

5. **Goal Journal**

A personalized tool for recording objectives, measuring progress, and reflecting on one's journey.

6. **Achievement Collage.**

An achievement collage is a visual depiction of accomplishments and victories, offering a concrete reflection of personal accomplishments. It provides a vital way to celebrate successes, boost self-esteem, and stay motivated.

7. **Winning Certificates**

A victory certificate is an official document that recognizes an individual or team's achievement in meeting a certain goal or milestone. While certificates are typically used in competitive situations such as contests, they may also be issued for a variety of accomplishments, such as successful completion of a training program or graduation.

8. **Appreciation for Self-Image and the Mirror**

The Appreciation of Self-Image and Mirror exercise is a simple yet effective activity that may help you feel more confident and accept yourself. Engaging in this practice might be useful if one is dealing with low self-esteem.

9. **Day of Positive Affirmations.**

Positive affirmations are a great tool for increasing self-esteem and improving general well-being. Using positive affirmations may be an effective way to improve one's life. When choosing affirmations, make sure they connect with you. Affirmations should be positive and encouraging, consistent with one's views and ideals.

10. Journal for Gratitude.

A thankfulness diary is a written document in which people write the things they are grateful for. It might be a simple notebook or a more detailed diary with questions and images. Setting out a certain time each day, even if it is just for a few minutes, to write in your diary is vital.

3.2 Strategies to Combat Self-Criticism

Self-criticism might seem to be motivational. It may have formerly served as a motivator and an effective instrument. However, if you're reading this, it's most certainly spread to other aspects of your life, causing more harm than good. Perhaps you believe that the inner critic voice will motivate you to study more, run faster, strive harder, perform better, etc. A motivational, encouraging tone is acceptable. The difficulty arises when we become unduly hard on ourselves. According to studies, self-criticism might diminish our chances of success and even halt our advancement. Critical self-talk may undermine motivation. It might cause procrastination and delay our progress. Negative self-talk drains our vitality and lowers our self-esteem. When you convince yourself that you will make mistakes, you are creating a self-fulfilling prophecy. "You didn't lick it off a stone" is an excellent Irish expression. It indicates that we are impacted by individuals around us, including those we grew up with and share genetics with. Does that sound like someone who tormented you in school? Does it make you think of an excessively critical relative or parent? Is your instructor harsh? Or someone you had a strained connection with?

Some young individuals discovered that when they were younger, their parents or teachers used harsh words to persuade them to accomplish things. These early encounters have an effect. We may believe that to complete tasks or fulfill the expectations of others, we must be very strict with ourselves. Internalizing is the process of borrowing and adopting another person's attitudes or critical words as our own. Sometimes, we have a valid cause for doing this. It could assist us in foreseeing attacks and avoiding them. Self-criticism may be created by attempting to protect oneself.

If this seems familiar, remember that you do not need or want an inner critic in your ear for the rest of your life. There are methods to lower the volume on it. Recognize its presence and origin. This should already be reducing its power.

Exercises to Deal with Self-Criticism

- **Phrases to tell yourself**

  You've undoubtedly heard of self-confidence mantras and positive affirmations. At first, they may seem ludicrous. But we all need them in our armory when self-critical comments start to bring us down.

  Try speaking the following words to yourself, starting with your name:

"You are doing your best."

"You're doing better than you think".

Replace ' should' with 'could'.

- **Replace ' should' with 'could'.**

'Should' is a restricting term that does not allow for context or compassion.

Consider this statement: "I should have prepared more for that exam." "I am such an idiot."

Changed to: "I could have prepared more for the exam." But I was exhausted from work the day before and couldn't stay up late to cram. Next time, I'll change shifts the day before a test."

- **Challenge the assertions.**

Self-critical sentiments are seldom accurate and often unduly harsh. When you hear these notions, halt and gently request proof.

If you think, "I'm a total idiot, and I will mess up this exam/game/project," say, "Let's look at the evidence." On a sheet of paper, put out all of the evidence you've got those points to failure.

On the other side of the page, detail all of the evidence against it. For example, you might include any additional tests you passed. Alternatively, you were assigned this project or placed in the team in the first place.

Now, sit back and consider the data on all sides. That should offer you a more sensible and clear perspective. If there are challenges ahead, determine how you will overcome them. If you're too overwhelmed to accomplish this exercise on your own, ask for support.

- **Take the power out of the voice.**

Don't tell your inner critic to shut up. Instead, modify the voice to that of an obnoxious cartoon character. Make it seem like Kermit the Frog or SpongeBob, and it will sound absurd. This makes it difficult to take what it says seriously.

Acknowledge perfectionism.

If you never attain your objectives and are dissatisfied with your accomplishments, you may be intentionally establishing unrealistic expectations. This is known as perfectionism. It is a sort of self-sabotage that may result in significant misery in the long term. Examine your self-imposed expectations. Are they realistic? Where do they come from? Try breaking them down and learning to live with variable expectations.

3.3 How to Build a Positive Body Image through Social Media

Help young people and children establish a good body image by confronting idealized pictures on social media platforms. Parents can empower them to place value on more than simply what they see in the mirror. Making kids aware of various body types might help them acquire a balanced perspective on body image. Many social networking programs have options for curating social feeds. This implies young people may conceal things they don't want to view while maintaining their social feeds.

Explore the suggestions listed below to get started.

- **Self-perception, body image, and identity**

  Young people consume a lot of stuff online, but not everything is as it seems, from deepfakes to body editors. However, it may be difficult for youngsters to determine what is and is not genuine online. As a result, people may attempt to live up to unachievable and edited ideals, making it difficult to maintain a good body image. When people strive to modify a portion of themselves to conform to that ideal, they may develop a negative self-image. This might have a significant influence on their overall health. One out of every ten girls aged 9 to 10 claim that being online makes them concerned about their physical shape or size, while 13% say it makes them the envy of others.

- **Tune, tweak, and filter**

  According to the Mental Health Foundation, around 37% of teenagers aged 13 to 19 were unhappy, and 31% were embarrassed of their body image. Further study by stem4 revealed that 3/4 of young people are dissatisfied with their appearance. As a result, when they use social media, they may be more prone to modify their images so that they look confident. However, they will continue to appear like themselves offline, making it more difficult to develop a good self-image.

- **Common editing applications**

  It's critical to have frequent, frank talks with your kid regarding their digital life. Inquire about the applications they're using, how they use them, and how it makes them feel. Being attentive to their digital environment may help them improve their self-image and well-being.

  Children who have a bad self-image may use editing applications to create a perfect representation of their looks. Some applications may only be used to adjust the colors or brightness of a photograph. However, programs that may alter the contour of a face or make a physique more muscular deserve additional consideration.

3.4 The Journey to Self-acceptance

Everyone has had the sensation of staring into the mirror and feeling dissatisfied with themselves for whatever reason. Perhaps the reason is that your eyes are not as close together as you would want. Perhaps you're upset with yourself for lately disappointing a buddy. You may want to lose a few pounds.

Our culture of comparison is much to blame for our self-deprecation. We see stunning sportsmen, actors, and models everywhere in the media. Our Darwinian inclinations would naturally advise us to evaluate ourselves against one another in an attempt to compete. However, this kind of competitiveness is unhealthy and eventually wears out. To be clear, appreciating who you are does not imply that you are incapable of growing personally. If you acted in a mean-spirited manner, make every effort to make things right while sticking to your principles. Go ahead and become blonde if you've always desired to and believe it would improve your self-esteem. Just watch out not to be too hard on yourself. People come and go from your life's tale. Although, in theory, everyone would support and be there for you, this isn't always the case. You alone are the one person you can be certain will always remain in your life. Although it may seem frightening, there is a benefit. You are the one who will always be there for you if you take care of yourself and appreciate who you are. Perhaps you're thinking it's easier said than done! Of course, you're correct. It is a lengthy procedure that is continuous. So, how can one go on a self-love journey? Here are some quick start suggestions:

1. Find the characteristics you appreciate rather than the ones that need improvement. Have you always despised the way your ears protruded? Stay away from it! What about that dimple you've always adored on your chin? Regarding that, smile! My friend suffered greatly from self-loathing and constantly evaluating herself against other people. When I asked her once what aspect of herself she enjoyed, she was unable to come up with anything. Although she is a lovely girl, she doesn't find anything appealing about the way she looks. If you catch yourself thinking in this way, try to modify it by developing yourself. All you need to do is learn to recognize your beauty. Even if you may not think of yourself as

conventionally attractive, you should accept the body you are in and stop trying to hate it!

2. Learn about who you are. You are probably a wonderful person! Perhaps, however, you've forgotten about it. I've discovered that keeping a diary is among the finest methods for understanding yourself. You discover a lot about your priorities when you allow your mind to run freely. Knowing that you can trust yourself with your ideas and secrets may also be freeing.

3. Give yourself a treat! Parks and Recreation was right when they said that it's necessary to reward oneself sometimes. Purchase a delightful chocolate bar, indulge in a soothing bath, or engage in any pleasurable activity. It's simple to be sucked into the hectic pace of family, school, and life overall, but always remember that you deserve to take a break and indulge in something enjoyable.

4. It takes time to learn to embrace who you are; it could take longer, based on where you start. Proceed at your speed, but keep in mind that wanting to be someone else won't get you anywhere. In the end, I hope being a teenager, you can come to accept and like who you are.

Chapter 4

Effective Communication and Relationship Management

Effective communication and relationship management are critical for teens as they negotiate adolescent obstacles and acquire vital social skills. This chapter teaches you all you need to know about effective communication and relationship management.

4.1 How to Use Assertiveness Training To Express Yourself Confidently

Assertive training is a kind of behavior therapy that teaches individuals how to stand up for themselves—or, to put it another way, empower themselves. It is an answer that strives to preserve an acceptable reaction in behavior while avoiding passivity and aggressiveness. Furthermore, it fosters justice and equality in human relationships by instilling a good sense of self-worth and respect for others. An assertive teen will preserve his or her boundaries while being respectful and compassionate to others. Purpose Assertiveness training is designed to educate individuals on effective skills for recognizing and acting on their objectives, needs, and views while staying respectful of others. Assertiveness training is a comprehensive technique that may be used in a variety of personal, healthcare, academic, and professional contexts. It is crucial to understand how to speak clearly and honestly since it leads to the improvement of connections with people around you (friends, family, and students).

An assertive person acts in his or her own best interests, defends himself or herself, communicates sentiments honestly, takes responsibility for oneself in interpersonal relationships, and makes decisions for oneself. The fundamental message delivered by an assertive individual is "I'm OK, and you're OK." An assertive individual is emotionally open, forthright, self-confident, and vocal. He/she feels secure and self-respectful both during and after his/her acts.

Building communication skills and confidence is critical for high school students as they manage adolescent issues and plan for the future. Teenagers are in the process of creating their identities and forming relationships, so now is an excellent time to teach assertiveness skills. Assertiveness enables pupils to successfully articulate their opinions, wants, and limits, resulting in both personal and academic achievement.

Assertiveness is sometimes misconstrued and associated with aggressiveness or passivity. It is critical to explain the difference. Assertiveness refers to the capacity to express oneself truthfully and boldly while respecting the rights and limits of others. It requires active listening skills, clear communication, and the capacity to negotiate and compromise. By teaching assertiveness, teachers can provide students with the skills they need to handle situations, advocate for themselves, and form healthy relationships. Effective communication requires a high level of confidence. When pupils lack self-confidence, they may fail to communicate adequately, resulting in misunderstandings and lost opportunities. Low self-confidence might also limit their capacity to articulate their demands and limits. By boosting students' confidence, we enable them to speak with conviction, clarity, and sincerity.

Approaches for Teaching Assertiveness in High School:

1. **Encourage self-awareness and reflection:**

   Help kids understand their own emotions, needs, and values. Journaling or self-assessment tasks might be useful for self-reflection.

2. **Teach excellent communication methods.**

   It includes active listening, empathy, and "I" statements. These abilities promote comprehension, assertiveness, and respect in conversation.

3. **Role-playing and scenario-based exercises:**

   Allow students to practice assertiveness in a safe atmosphere. Role-playing situations might assist children in gaining confidence and forceful communication abilities.

4. **Create a friendly and inclusive classroom atmosphere.**

   Create a safe atmosphere in which kids may express themselves. Encourage peer support and cooperation to help create a culture that values boldness and open communication.

5. **Adding Social Emotional Learning (SEL) to Assertiveness Training:**

   Social Emotional Learning (SEL) is an essential component in teaching assertiveness skills. SEL focuses on the development of self-awareness, self-management, and interpersonal skills. Integrating SEL exercises into assertiveness training helps students acquire the emotional intelligence required for successful, assertive communication.

6. **Addressing Challenges and Eliminating Barriers:**

   Teaching assertiveness skills in your high school may present difficulties, such as student opposition or a lack of support from parents or authorities. To overcome these obstacles, it is critical to persevere and argue for the benefits of assertiveness training. Providing continual assistance and tools may also help the students conquer their internal obstacles.

4.2 How to Handle Relationships and peer Pressure

Pressure is a natural and difficult aspect of life for everyone. However, how we approach it differs greatly from person to person. Peer pressure, in particular, may be very difficult to cope with throughout adolescence. Teenagers seek to satisfy their classmates in order to fit in. They are afraid of distancing themselves; therefore, they don't say no.

It's critical to remember that most peer pressure isn't how it seems in films or television programs. These programs depict classmates encouraging vulnerable teenagers, "Do this if you're going to be one of us," or "If you don't do this, you're a loser." In the actual world, peer pressure may be considerably more subtle. It is motivated by an urge to feel "normal," which intensifies throughout puberty. As a result, we assist our children in defining their beliefs and considering what they want for themselves in order to better prepare them to navigate adolescent culture. Parents may encourage kids to pursue their views and emotions while yet feeling like they fit in. Teens may learn to deal with and resist peer pressure if they are equipped with certain abilities. We can teach teenagers how to make a difference by examining the following techniques.

Strategies for Teaching Teens to Deal with Peer Pressure.

- **Have the courage to walk away.**

  We all want to be liked by our peers; therefore, it might be difficult to be the sole one saying "no" when confronted with peer pressure. You must educate them to believe in themselves. You may do this by role modeling confidence and appreciating their excellent decisions. By doing so, their inner power will allow them to remain steadfast in their emotions. A strong sense of self-worth will enable them to act in accordance with their beliefs. That same confidence leads them to be less afraid of failure. It's a mix that allows individuals to reject peer pressure while yet having the fortitude to walk away. They will understand that, even if they "fail" in front of their peers, they will ultimately achieve.

- **Look for Positive Peer "Partners".**

If your kids lack the confidence to walk away on their own, urge them to seek out a classmate or buddy who shares their feelings in a specific scenario. If they are being pressured to skip class, are tempted to use drugs, or are concerned about classmates harassing another student, having a buddy who is equally prepared to say "no" helps them resist that temptation.

- **Set limits and say no.**

Teens dislike having to say no to their friends or classmates. They are concerned that doing so may jeopardize an otherwise positive connection. As parents, you establish safe boundaries for your teenagers. You must also teach kids to realize that saying no is acceptable in certain situations. Using illegal drugs or driving a person who has been drinking are examples of situations in which they must say no. For example, if your kids are uneasy attending parties where their parents are not present, educate them on how to gently refuse a party invitation while avoiding hurt feelings. If they are pushed by friends to smoke cigarettes, they may answer, "No thanks." I am not into it. "I feel sick just being around smoke." Although we desire our children to be polite, our daughters must understand that saying "No!" may also be the proper thing to do. When individuals learn to establish their boundaries, they will feel more in control in a variety of circumstances throughout their lives.

- **Teach teenagers to stay away.**

Have you heard the classic joke about the patient who says, "Doc, my arm aches when I do this!" The doctor responds, "Then don't do that!" That goofy joke has some important knowledge. If your adolescents feel pressured by their classmates to do things, they know are bad, encourage them to avoid stressful circumstances in the first place. If they know that a gang of teenagers is looking for trouble, they should avoid going out with them. If kids know a corner is unsafe, go around the block the other way.

Because shunning pleasure or peers entirely is never a good idea, we should encourage young people to seek out compatible peers or fellow students who avoid dangerous or imprudent circumstances.

- **Develop Decision-Making Skills. When it comes to peer pressure.**

It is critical to empower teenagers to make daily choices for themselves. If parents constantly make decisions for their teenagers, they transmit the message that they are unable to. Teens can only genuinely improve their decision-making abilities if they get the opportunity to put them into practice! As kids make their own decisions, they will feel better about their choices and may be more inclined to do the right thing.

- **Ask questions and consider the consequences.**

  When in a difficult circumstance, asking questions aloud to a buddy or a group of peers may help you gain support and relieve stress. For example, if kids are being persuaded to shoplift, tell them what they may ask their classmates. "Who thought it was a good idea? Whose decision was this? Why would we want to do this? "Won't we be arrested if we get caught?" Hearing repercussions spoken out might also cause peers to reflect and even change their thoughts about the exact thing they were urging others to undertake.

- **Speak with a trustworthy adult if they feel pressured.**

  If peer pressure is still too much for your kids, let them know they don't have to cope with it alone. Remind them that you're there for them. If they seem to be unable to approach you for the time being, let them know that it is equally OK to seek counsel from a trustworthy adult other than you. Extended family, teachers, pastors, counselors, and coaches are all valuable resources. They may provide advice and assistance in dealing with high-pressure circumstances.

- **Teach Teens Coping Strategies.**

  It does not take long for youngsters to understand that life is full of options. When our children reach puberty, they understand that making decisions may be difficult and stressful. Listening to their intuition, concentrating on their strengths, talking through problems, and adopting relaxation techniques are all examples of coping mechanisms that may assist in managing stress. Teaching and modeling coping methods can help kids make better choices under stressful and hard circumstances that are often associated with peer pressure.

- **Go ahead and "blame the parents".**

Provide your adolescents with an excuse to cope with peer pressure if other methods fail. Let them know you're OK with their using you as an exit. Consider the effect of telling pals, "If I skip school today, my mother will punish me for the next three months!" or "My father said I couldn't attend the party. If I do and get caught, I'll lose my driving rights."

- **It's Okay to make mistakes.**

Everyone makes errors. If their short error of judgment does not jeopardize their safety or morals, attempt to remain cool. Have a decent conversation when some time has elapsed. It should be a nonjudgmental discourse. If possible, relate an example of a mistake you made when you were younger and explain what you learned from it. That fairness will motivate students to make good decisions if they are presented with a similar peer circumstance in the future. Your adaptability in these areas will also help you to take harder positions in areas that threaten their safety or morals.

Being there for teenagers when they encounter the problems of peer pressure may have a huge impact. Our tweens and adolescents are listening to us, even if it doesn't always seem that way. Teens who are equipped with a range of communication methods are more likely to make sound judgments when confronted with peer pressure. These are skills that will help kids not just get through difficult circumstances now, but also later in life.

4.3 How to Understand and Improve Family Relationships

It's crucial to enter the situation prepared if you want to confront your problem head-on and speak with your family members or members about it. Concentrate on a single issue that you want to tackle, such as a time limit that is too harsh or pressure from school. Have your objective in mind when you frame the talk with them.

- **Learn about their viewpoint.**

This is not a lecture you are giving your family member; rather, this is a discussion. Give their opinions your entire attention, and maybe they'll return the favor. Even if you disagree with someone's viewpoint, you may still respect and affirm it. Keep in mind that your family member is a human being with ideas and emotions of their own, which may influence how they behave. Investigate it thoroughly to come up with a solution that benefits you both.

Teens may have social, political, or religious views and feelings that differ from their parents, which can also lead to tensions." "Parents who want to give their teens the right boundaries but also give them more independence and freedom as they get closer to adulthood sometimes find themselves in conflict."

- **Communicate clearly and honestly.**

Generally, you want to ensure that your argument is strong when speaking with parents or guardians. You may do it by focusing just on certain circumstances and the feelings they evoke in you. You can debate with generalizations (e.g., "You never trust me!"), but not with facts.

"When you read through my messages yesterday, I was incredibly offended. I felt as if I had no control over the discussions, I had with myself.

Here, the "I" words are crucial. You are communicating to your family members how they have affected you by speaking from your own experience, even if they may not always be aware of it.

- **Steer clear of it while you can.**

When you need a break from your family, take advantage of the opportunity to just go for a stroll or visit a friend's home. If your family is less lenient when it comes to your travels, look for ways to leave the home that they would support, such as joining an after-school activity or sports team.

Try your best to avoid getting into arguments with troublesome family members if you are unable to stay away from them. Determine any trigger issues that might elicit a negative reaction and make an effort to avoid them. Therefore, maybe keep your ideas for when you're with your pals if your father gets agitated every time you bring up politics.

- **When you are unable to redirect.**

Redirect the discussion or your behavior if you find yourself in a difficult position with your family. Here are a few methods to follow:

Make lighthearted remarks. Make jokes about the situation by joking that you're always going to be single if your family member is persistently pressuring you about your dating life.

- **Go off-topic.**

Ask your family members a completely different inquiry, such as how they prepared the dish you're eating if they start making fun of a social cause you care about at dinner.

- **Make a helping offer.**

Offer to load the dishwasher for your family members if they are extremely worried about all the dirty dishes in the sink to avoid giving them a lecture.

4.3 Conflict Resolution Strategies For Teenagers

As teenagers negotiate their social contacts and relationships, disputes are unavoidable. Conflict may be unpleasant and emotionally draining, but it doesn't have to be. Developing conflict resolution skills may help youngsters handle problems constructively and peacefully, resulting in stronger and better relationships. In this topic, we will look at some successful dispute resolution tactics for teens. Educate teens with practical advice and recommendations for improving their conflict resolution skills and preventing disagreements from escalating. Conflict resolution is an important ability for teens to learn as they negotiate the various social and personal problems that come up during this time of life. Teenagers may learn to handle disagreements calmly and constructively by practicing good communication, empathy, active listening, and problem-solving strategies.

Teenagers should realize that conflict is a normal aspect of life and that there are healthy methods to address it. Teenagers may avoid increasing arguments and foster healthy relationships by staying assertive and using proactive techniques such as conflict resolution activities and peer mediation. As kids grow, they will face conflict in a variety of situations, including school, job, and personal relationships. By developing long-term conflict resolution skills, students may have the confidence and capacity to manage these circumstances with grace and diplomacy. Conflict is an unavoidable aspect of human contact, and teens are no different. Conflict occurs when two or more people disagree on their perspectives, needs, beliefs, or values. It may cause unpleasant feelings, tension, and even violence if not addressed constructively. Teenage conflict resolution requires effective communication abilities. Clear and courteous communication may assist them in determining the fundamental cause of the issue, finding common ground, and reaching a mutually acceptable resolution.

Peer mediation is a successful technique for dispute resolution in schools that includes trained student mediators resolving problems with their peers. This program seeks to enable students to recognize and address problems, as well as to build communication and problem-solving skills that will allow them to resolve disagreements peacefully. Teenagers who get peer mediation training may gain significant dispute-resolution skills that will improve not just their academic environment but also their social and personal lives. Active listening, problem-solving, empathy, and communication are examples of these abilities. Peer mediation programs have various advantages, including enhancing the school environment, lowering disciplinary measures, and cultivating a good, empathetic culture. They also provide a secure, impartial environment for pupils to express their worries and sentiments.

Conflict Resolution Practices for Teenagers

Conflict resolution skills are critical for teens as they manage the intricacies of relationships and societal dynamics. Engaging in conflict resolution activities allows youngsters to practice these skills in a safe and supportive setting. Here are some useful conflict resolution practices for teenagers:

1. Role-playing conflict scenarios might help youngsters develop critical thinking skills for real-life circumstances. They may take turns playing various roles and devising solutions that benefit everyone involved.

2. Team-building activities improve teens' communication and teamwork abilities, which are crucial for successful dispute resolution. Examples include constructing a spaghetti and marshmallow tower or completing a ropes course.

3. Board games, like Diplomacy or Settlers of Catan, may help build dispute resolution skills. Teenagers may practice making compromises and finding mutually beneficial solutions.

4. Encourage teens to journal their thoughts and experiences to improve conflict resolution skills and communication. They may also write about disputes they've watched or experienced and how they might have been handled better.

5. Debriefing exercises: After resolving a disagreement, teens may reflect on what worked well and areas for improvement. This may help individuals improve their conflict resolution skills and gain confidence in their capacity to manage future disputes.

Overall, conflict resolution exercises may be an effective way for teens to improve their problem-solving and communication abilities. Encouraging kids to participate in these activities might help them become better at resolving disagreements in their social and personal lives.

Tips for Effective Conflict Resolution.

Conflicts are an unavoidable part of life, but understanding how to settle them successfully may help us enhance our relationships and save unneeded stress. Here are a few conflict resolution techniques to help teens manage their problems calmly and productively:

1. Actively listen to the other person without interrupting or judgment. To demonstrate your understanding of their point of view, paraphrase and summarize their arguments.

2. Communicate assertively: Express your wants and emotions clearly and politely, using "I" phrases rather than criticizing or accusing others. Avoid criticizing the other person's character or making generalizations.

3. Identify common ground. Look for areas of collaboration or shared aims to use as a beginning point for resolving the disagreement. Concentrate on the issue, not the individual.

4. Brainstorm conflict resolution strategies and possible implications: Evaluate the benefits and drawbacks of each option before deciding which one best satisfies the requirements of all parties.

5. Use humor: Bringing lightheartedness to a tough situation may reduce tension and provide a new viewpoint.

Remember that the goal of conflict resolution is to find a solution that is agreeable to all parties. Use these conflict resolution suggestions, together with critical thinking skills, to settle disagreements constructively and productively.

Chapter 5

Goal Setting and Future Planning

The teenage years are exciting times in life, full of goals and ambitions. But having dreams by themselves won't get you there. The secret to making your aspirations come true is to set objectives. You will discover how to prepare for the future and make goals in this chapter.

5.1 Exercises to Explore Aspirations and Dreams

Set wise objectives, and you'll carve out a clear road to realizing your aspirations. Some wise objectives that teens might establish to realize their desires are discussed in this topic.

- **Academic Prominence**

  Achieving academic achievement is essential for both personal development and prospects. A major factor in determining your knowledge, abilities, and future opportunities is your education. Establishing academic excellence objectives will help you get closer to realizing your aspirations for college. Start by evaluating your current academic situation and pinpointing any areas that need improvement. To improve your grades in difficult topics, develop better study habits, and take an active role in class discussions, set specific academic objectives. To help you stay focused and monitor your progress, break these objectives down into smaller, more doable activities. The development of efficient study strategies is necessary for academic achievement. Make it your mission to create a regular study schedule that suits your preferred method of learning. Establish a calm and orderly study area, set up certain times of the day for studying, and make use of a variety of tools, including study groups, internet resources, and textbooks. Recall that achieving success requires not only putting in the work but also using useful techniques like practicing problem-solving, summarizing notes, and routinely revisiting the content.

Seek chances for intellectual development outside of the classroom as well. Make it your mission to learn more about topics that interest you, join groups or contests at school, or do independent study. Getting involved in your topic of interest outside of the classroom expands your knowledge and shows that you are enthusiastic about and committed to your academic goals. Maintaining a healthy balance between your academics and other facets of your life is crucial when aiming for academic success. Make self-care a priority, keep up good connections, and participate in extracurricular activities that feed your hobbies. Recall that being academically excellent involves more than simply getting good marks; it also involves developing a lifelong love of learning and gaining useful abilities.

- **Personal Growth**

Putting money into your personal development is an empowering adventure that helps you reach your greatest potential and become the person you've always wanted to be. Establishing personal development objectives is crucial for developing your talents, fostering your interests, and boosting your self-esteem.

Find out what aspects of personal growth speak to you first. Make it a point to read literature that will increase your horizons and your knowledge. Reading introduces you to new concepts, people, and civilizations while fostering empathy and critical thinking abilities.

Furthermore, establish objectives to acquire a new skill or engage in a pastime that complements your interests. Engaging in creative endeavors such as painting, computing, music theory, sports, or art classes fosters your imagination, self-expression, and self-control. Developing one's self-confidence is yet another essential component of personal growth. Make it your mission to take on difficulties that will force you to go outside your comfort zone. This might include giving speeches in front of an audience, joining a debating group, or taking part in leadership activities.

Accept setbacks as teaching opportunities and use them to become more resilient and powerful. Be in the company of uplifting people and look for mentoring or advice from those who can encourage and inspire you.

Furthermore, developing excellent communication skills is a component of personal growth. Establish objectives to enhance your speaking, listening, and writing communication skills. Participate in writing contests, public speaking classes, or school newspaper membership to hone your communication skills. Meaningful relationships may be forged both professionally and personally via effective communication.

Setting objectives for personal development will result in ongoing progress and self-improvement since personal development is a lifetime endeavor. Accept the chance to reflect on yourself, acknowledge your accomplishments, and be willing to modify your life objectives when circumstances change. You may invest in your success, happiness, and contentment by investing in your personal growth.

- **Optimal Way of Living**

One of the most important things for teenagers to focus on is maintaining a healthy lifestyle since it fosters well-being and lays the groundwork for a happy and prosperous adult life. By prioritizing your mental and physical well-being, you can make sure you have the stamina, determination, and energy to follow your aspirations.

Start by deciding how you want to use regular exercise in your routine. Try to get in at least 30 minutes of exercise most days of the week. Whether it's swimming, dancing, jogging, or playing sports, choose something you want to do. Frequent exercise not only increases physical fitness but also elevates mood, eases stress, and sharpens cognitive abilities. A healthy diet should be your objective in addition to exercise. Make an effort to include a range of entire grains, vegetables, fruits, lean meats, and healthy fats in your meals. Steer clear of processed meals, sugary snacks, and sugary drinks in excess.

Establish clear objectives, including increasing your water intake, carrying a nutritious lunch, and preparing wholesome meals at home. Keep in mind that even modest, long-lasting dietary adjustments may have a big influence on your general health and well-being. Maintaining your emotional well-being is just as crucial. Establish objectives for yourself to practice stress-reduction methods like deep breathing, meditation, or relaxing hobbies. Make self-care routines a priority, such as getting adequate sleep, meditating, and asking friends, family, or experts for help. Keep in mind that leading a healthy lifestyle involves taking care of your mental, physical, and emotional health.

You are investing in yourself and making sure you have the energy and vigor to zealously pursue your aspirations by making goals for a healthy lifestyle. Accept the power of consistent exercise, a healthy diet, and self-care routines to provide the groundwork for a fulfilling and well-rounded existence. Your most valuable resource is your health, which you can take good care of to get the most out of every aspect of your life.

- **Prudent Budgeting**

Being financially responsible as a teenager prepares you for success in the future and gives you the ability to make informed financial choices. Establishing objectives in this area guarantees that you possess the know-how and abilities to handle finances well.

Set aside some of your income as your first aim. Set aside a certain percentage or amount for savings, whether from a side hustle, an allowance, part-time work, or other sources. Early adoption of this practice fosters discipline and creates a safety net for finances. Create a bank account or a savings account to make things simpler. Establish savings objectives for both immediate requirements, like buying a desired item, and long-term objectives, like funding a college education or making investments in the future. Establish objectives to make and stick to a budget in addition to saving. Keep a close eye on your earnings and outlays to have a clear picture of where your money is going. Set up money for both luxuries like entertainment or personal goods and necessities like transportation, food, and schooling costs. Knowing that you have sufficient funds to cover all of your necessary purchases can alleviate your mind.

Make careful to discern between necessities and desires to make wise financial decisions. Establish objectives to reduce wasteful spending and discover methods of saving money, such as price comparison, discount shopping, or looking into more affordable options. This will assist you in avoiding requesting financial assistance that can result in unwelcome debt.

Moreover, establish objectives to master the fundamentals of personal finance. Learn about things like investing, credit ratings, and interest rates. Think about establishing objectives to study books or enroll in online courses on personal finance.

Gaining an understanding of these ideas will enable you to manage credit, plan for the future, and make wise borrowing and saving choices. Look for ways to make money via extracurricular activities or business endeavors; they may help you become financially independent and impart important skills like accountability, time management, and work ethic.

- **Digital Accountability**

Being responsible online is essential for your reputation and general well-being in the modern digital world. Establishing objectives for digital responsibility guarantees secure online navigation, privacy protection, and thoughtful technology usage.

Establish objectives first to keep a favorable digital presence. Make it a point to consider what you're posting before doing so since your online presence matters. Think about the possible repercussions of your online behavior, including the comments, information, and pictures you publish.

Additionally, make plans for protecting your online security and privacy. Examine and update your internet accounts' and social media networks' privacy settings. Aim to generate secure, one-of-a-kind passwords for every account.

Be careful while disclosing personal information online and be on the lookout for any phishing or scam efforts. Make objectives for yourself to become knowledgeable about online safety procedures and dangers to protect your digital identity. You may avoid such dangers and guarantee a safer online experience by taking proactive measures to safeguard your privacy.

Establish objectives to improve your ability to think critically while reading internet stuff. It's critical to distinguish trustworthy sources from false information or fake news due to the abundance of information available online. Aim to confirm the information before disseminating it and consider the reliability of the sources. Look for trustworthy websites and fact-checking groups to make sure the material you come across is true.

Make an effort to have a good digital effect, safeguard your privacy, and keep yourself educated while using the internet. By establishing objectives for digital responsibility, you may use technology's potential while keeping a positive and harmonious connection with the digital realm.

- **Time Management**

Being able to manage your time well is essential if you want to maximize your days, accomplish your objectives, and have a positive work-life balance. Establishing objectives for time management enables you to prioritize work, maintain organization, accomplish your objectives, and increase productivity.

To start, make objectives so that you may create a daily schedule that suits you. Establish the best times to study, do homework, participate in extracurricular activities, and unwind. To make sure you get adequate sleep, set clear objectives for when you should get up and go to bed each day. Establishing a schedule for your day helps you feel more in control and makes you less tired of making decisions, which frees up time for crucial responsibilities.

Establish objectives to improve your ability to prioritize and plan. Use digital tools to help you keep organized or set particular objectives to make lists of things to accomplish. Divide more complex jobs into smaller, more doable segments, and set reasonable due dates. Sort jobs into high- and low-priority categories, paying special attention to the former. You may reduce procrastination and guarantee that each work gets enough time by establishing objectives to efficiently plan and prioritize.

Additionally, make objectives to maximize your productivity and reduce distractions. Establish objectives to efficiently manage distractions, such as social media, excessive alerts, or ineffective routines.

For instance, you may choose certain times for social media monitoring and turn off alerts when concentrating on work. To establish a distraction-free atmosphere that is beneficial to studying or working, think about defining objectives. You may increase the quality of your work and your ability to concentrate by establishing objectives to reduce distractions and create a productive atmosphere.

Time is an important resource that is irreversibly lost once used. You are investing in your general well-being and productivity when you establish time management objectives. Accept the value of setting priorities, preparing ahead, and avoiding distractions. You can do more in less time, lower your stress level, and have more chances to engage in leisure activities and follow your interests when you practice disciplined time management. It's a wise objective to pursue.

5.2 How to Set Achievable Goals

With a little bit of luck and a lot of effort, goals provide us with something to strive for, a purpose to keep us motivated, and an occasion to celebrate.

For young individuals, learning how to create objectives is an essential ability. It isn't easy to travel without knowing where you are going, after all. Teens who set goals are better able to stay focused on the path to their objectives, establish plans, manage their time and resources, and recognize when they may need assistance.

Learning how to make goals is beneficial for teenagers in many ways, including:

- Reaching the intended outcome, which is the ultimate aim of every goal!

- gaining confidence as you go through the process.

- recognizing and enhancing their work ethic, discovering the most effective ways to inspire them, strengthening their resilience in the face of setbacks, and knowing when to seek assistance or support.

Teens who have objectives are better able to implement their ideas. They will benefit greatly from these abilities on a personal, academic, and professional level. Setting goals is simple, but coming up with a plan of action to get there may be difficult. Writing goal statements that contain the precise actions you must do to reach the objective is possible with SMART goals.

An acronym called "SMART" may be used to direct the goal-setting process. (And the good news is that SMART objectives apply to all age groups!)

Objectives need to be:

- Specific: The objective should be sufficiently defined to enable teenagers to concentrate their efforts and make clear the actions they want to take. It should not be too broad.

- Measurable: The objective has to be quantifiable. They see changes when they can quantify a goal. Additionally, youth will be more successful and able to remain on course.

- Achievable: The objective needs to be reachable. They won't stick with a goal they establish for themselves if it is too difficult for them to achieve. If they are significant, attainable objectives aid in the development of attitudes, aptitudes, and talents.

- Realistic: The objective ought to be doable. Raising the bar will result in a fulfilling accomplishment. There must be some work involved.

- Time-bound: The objective must be completed within a realistic time frame. Short-term objectives may be divided into manageable tasks that can be completed quickly. Over an extended duration, long-term objectives may be divided into time-based short-term objectives.

Teens should make sure their objective fits the above criteria and is SMART while they are thinking about what they want to accomplish. It's then time to think about how and when they will measure the aim.

How to Teach Teens to Set Goals

Get ready, set, go! After learning about SMART goals and the advantages of goal-setting for teenagers, consider the following five suggestions for helping kids create goals:

- **Set an example for goal-setting in your own life.**

One of the most obvious methods to introduce goal-setting to your adolescent is to show them that you establish objectives and work toward achieving them. Throughout the process, be honest with them about any changes or failures, as well as the efforts you're making to reach your objective. These talks may be informal, but they help your adolescent understand that things need time and effort to achieve by demonstrating the amount of work you put in that they might not be aware of. An additional advantage is that your kid could serve as a cheerleader or accountability partner for you while you work toward your objective. Creating a plan to find a new job; establishing a new healthy habit, like getting enough sleep or journaling; adhering to a budget to save toward something; leading or assisting in neighborhood or community initiatives; working toward participating in a larger event, like training for a 5K run; learning a new skill; and making time for friends, family, and neighbors are a few examples of goal-setting that adults can model for teens.

- **Create a strategy.**

Your kid should create a strategy for reaching their goal after deciding on one to strive toward. Putting it in writing often helps your adolescent feel more accountable and makes it seem true. A target plan needs to state the following:

1. What the objective is.

2. The intended outcome, quantifiable progress markers, actions to be taken in between each of those markers, and a timeline for completing the stages and reaching the final objective

3. Any accountability they desire (and from whom); how would they like to monitor their development?

- **Allow teenagers to take the lead.**

  Teens who set their objectives, make their plans, and pursue them are the ones with the greatest outcomes. Experiences that are self-driven are often the most fulfilling and inspiring, and they provide a wealth of learning opportunities. For teenagers who want to be independent and will be in a few years, this is extremely important. Allow them to lead the goal-setting process, from selecting an objective to pursuing it (and changing course when things don't go according to plan). They will gain experiences and life lessons along the road, and ideally, they will understand the joy that comes from a job well done when their objective is accomplished. Lean out and let adolescents lead the way, but as their support system, periodically inquire about how their aim is going or offer to listen when they have a setback.

- **Celebrate every accomplishment of a goal.**

  It is more vital than ever to take time to rejoice in a hectic society where we often move quickly. As the adult in their lives, make sure your adolescent knows how to celebrate a job well done. Set an example for them by doing so yourself every day.

Since SMART objectives include quantifiable benchmarks, make sure to recognize and commemorate each milestone reached. When a long-term goal is reached, throw a huge party.

Students might set short-term objectives such as these:

- Establish and maintain a new routine, like working out or journaling.

- Establish a nighttime and morning routine that will help you succeed.

- Make a savings deposit.

- Clean and arrange your spaces.

- Locate a mentor who can assist in putting you in touch with opportunities.

- Put in more study time to improve your exam or topic score.

- Complete a certain number of books that month or that year.

- Spend a day helping out in your neighborhood or school.

- Write a cover letter.

- Experiment with a new pastime, sport, or talent to determine whether it's something you want to pursue.

Long-term objectives for students may look something like this:

- Aim for a timely high school graduation.

- Commit to a long-term project, such as organizing a team or community event or beginning a new endeavor, like learning to sew or creating a podcast.

- To get a license, prepare for and sit for a driving test.

- Acquire a new language.

- Consider taking up a work shadowing, part-time employment, or internship as a means of exploring potential career paths.

- Make plans for life beyond high school graduation and submit college applications.

5.3 How to Make Informed and Thoughtful Choices

Every day, teenagers have to make choices that might change their lives. However, most teenagers never get instruction on how to make wise judgments. Because of this, some teenagers find it difficult to make judgments like: Should I get a job? When a buddy offers me a cigarette, what should I say? Do I approach someone to go on a date? Is engaging in sexual activity acceptable? Making wise decisions as a teen may help position them for success in the future. Furthermore, youth with strong decision-making abilities are better able to control their stress levels.

- **Provide Direction**

  Encouraging your child to make wise choices requires giving them plenty of direction without going overboard. When it's needed, provide advice, but don't be scared to take a backseat and allow your adolescent to make errors. Natural consequences may sometimes teach us important life lessons. Just remember to be there for your adolescent when they fall short. Encourage them to talk about how to make better decisions in the future and help them learn from their failures.

- **Determine the Issue**

Teenagers may choose to ignore issues or place the blame elsewhere. Teens may claim that since their math instructor doesn't explain the homework, they are failing the subject. Alternatively, individuals can put off finishing their assignments because they find the mountain of work, they've been putting off worrying too much.

Thus, it's crucial to occasionally assist your adolescent in articulating the issue. Start a dialogue with your teenager and solicit their opinion by asking queries such as "What do you feel is going on here?"

- **List All of Your Options**

Help your child recognize their possibilities. Teens often believe that there are only one or two ways to solve an issue. But given enough time and support, they can often provide a lengthy list of original ideas. Encourage them to jot down as many as they can, listing each one so they can later study it.

Encourage your child to name as many options as they can, even if they don't seem like good ideas.

- **Examine the Benefits and Drawbacks**

After your adolescent has a list of choices, ask them to outline any possible advantages and disadvantages for each. They can determine which alternative could be the greatest option by outlining the benefits and drawbacks.

Discuss how emotions may influence choices significantly. They could misjudge the danger out of enthusiasm or fear while attempting something new.

Teens may approach an issue logically by outlining the benefits and drawbacks of many solutions in writing, as opposed to making a choice only based on feelings.

Have your child decide which option appears the greatest. Try to encourage your child to choose their own, but feel free to provide suggestions and direction as needed.

Assure your child that making a decision isn't necessarily a terrible idea. There are advantages and disadvantages to choosing between two reputable universities, yet both can be worthwhile. So, while having to make a decision might be unpleasant, it could be a nice issue to have.

- **Make a Strategy to Proceed**

After your child has weighed the advantages and disadvantages of their selections, discuss the next steps. Decide what actions they should take next. Additionally, discuss how to assess their decision. It's critical to assess if it was beneficial or whether they erred. Analyzing the effectiveness of their decision may teach them valuable lessons and help them make even better choices in the future.

5.4 How to Deal with Uncertainty and Change

Life is full of uncertainty, and the epidemic has made it harder for individuals of all ages to deal with the unknown. However, the psychological toll that COVID-19 has had on youth has been very challenging. Indeed, according to a recent poll, 64% of teenagers think that the Covid-19 experience will have a long-term effect on the mental health of their generation. Teens' need for assistance with accepting uncertainty is a recurring topic in our present therapy practice.

What does it mean to put up with ambiguity?

Certain individuals handle uncertainty better than others. The capacity to deal with or tolerate uncertain circumstances is known as uncertainty tolerance. A person who has a high threshold for uncertainty is more adept at adjusting to uncontrollable circumstances. When presented with unfamiliar conditions, those who have a low threshold for uncertainty are more prone to exhibit feelings of worry, tension, and depression.

Strategies for Dealing with Uncertainty and Change

In therapy, a parent should share with the teenagers they work with the good news: you can develop your ability to tolerate uncertainty in the same way that you can grow your muscles. Some strategies for young people to build their muscles of uncertainty tolerance are outlined below.

- **Put acceptance into practice.**

Though painful, emotions cannot harm you. We educate them that embracing uncertainty and not running away from the associated pain is the best way to deal with it. Eliminating or avoiding pain or stress is a common reaction. Teens who practice mindfulness are better able to focus on being mindfully in the present moment without trying to alter it. They become more naturally aware and have a far better capacity to withstand any unpleasant feeling, including uncertainty, when they practice mindfulness techniques.

- **Work on the opposite action.**

A Dialectical Behavioral Therapy (DBT) technique called "opposite action" involves purposefully acting in the opposite way from how we usually handle our emotions. In this setting, it is instructed to teenagers on how to identify the actions that they would most likely do in the event of emotional distress. Retrenchment to seeking comfort about the epidemic via news articles, internet reporting, and social media is a typical reaction we hear. Teens who engage in these behaviors usually do it in their bedrooms by themselves. It is encouraged to practice opposing action by acting in a way that conflicts with their desire to always be connected to the news. Leaving the phone at home and going for a block stroll is one example of this. Alternatively, switching off the phone whether viewing a movie or reading a book.

- **Recognize and question automatic thinking patterns.**

It's possible for us to automatically think negatively when faced with uncertainty. These kinds of beliefs often fit into many categories that we call cognitive distortions. Cognitive distortions are automatic, often unreliable, and unfavorably biased methods of thinking. Parents should educate teenagers in cognitive restructuring so they can recognize, question, and change their harmful ideas.

- **Concentrate on what you can manage.**

List all the things that are causing you anxiety or tension. Next, divide the list into two columns: those that you can manage and those that you cannot. For instance, we have no control over when sports or schools will return, but we do have control over how we socialize with friends and exercise in a secure environment. We may go on with the things we can control and strive to accept the things we cannot by adopting a solution-focused attitude. Teens who are more adept at handling uncertainty will be less likely to suffer from anxiety and depression, which will make it easier for them to handle stress as well as the inevitable stress they will face in the future.

Chapter 6

Interactive and Reflective Exercises

Getting in touch with your emotions and thoughts may be facilitated by reflecting on relationships, everyday events, and personal beliefs. It can result in more mental tranquility. All of the interactive and reflective exercises that teens should be familiar with are covered in this chapter.

6.1 Guided Prompts for Self-reflection

One of the finest methods to support children (particularly teenagers) in developing self-worth and confidence is via journaling. It also teaches them to reflect on their lives, gives them stability, and naturally fosters creativity. It's more crucial than ever to examine your emotions and deliberately express them. For teenagers who already have a lot on their minds, this is not the simplest assignment. For this reason, we have compiled a list of some thoughtful journaling topics for teenagers that will aid in their self-expression, understanding of their emotions, and, most importantly, self-expression.

1. What gives you a sense of strength?

2. What calms you down?

3. What gives you a sense of mastery?

4. What is your strategy for motivating oneself to attempt something new?

5. Based on your requirements, what decision can you make this week?

6. If changing your perspective doesn't work for you, how do you do it?

7. What is your recharging strategy?

8. How are you going to honor yourself today?

9. How does your current situational best look?

10. What encourages you to become more mindful and slow down?

11. One year from now, what is anything you can accomplish that you didn't think you could do?

12. What is your desired outcome and why?

13. How can you prioritize your needs without feeling bad about it?

14. How do you go about accepting yourself?

15. How do you avoid distractions and maintain focus?

16. How much do you trust your ability to make important decisions?

17. How do you draw boundaries, so you don't take on the tension and feelings of other people?

18. How do you make the most of your alone time?

19. How can you tell when burnout is approaching?

20. How do you express your emotions to those who are close to you?

21. When other people succeed, how can you turn your jealousy into happiness?

22. In what ways do you speak out for yourself?

23. When you make a mistake, how do you grant yourself forgiveness?

24. When you need assistance or support, how do you ask for it?

25. How do you show yourself compassion and self-love?

26. In a challenging circumstance, how do you relieve tension?

27. How do you intentionally spend more time with people?

28. How do you accept who you really are, even when it doesn't appear like what other people think you should?

29. How do you establish and maintain your boundaries?

30. What fresh chances have arisen as a result of obstacles you have overcome?

6.2 How to Use Art, Music, and Writing for Emotional Relief

The easy stages are to write down your top ideas and have a brainstorming session to release emotional stress. It's important to pay attention to your inner voice and to embrace all of your feelings and ideas with love. The ability to express and let go of all of one's emotions and anxieties via art, music, and writing therapy is its biggest advantage.

Emotional Relief Through Art Therapy

Teenagers and young adults dealing with a variety of issues, including grief, family dissolution, low self-esteem, anxiety, bad mood, behavioral or social issues, or issues related to abuse, neglect, or trauma, may find relief via art therapy. Numerous studies have shown that working directly with art supplies, creating a meaningful art object, channeling emotions into a piece of work, and interacting with a therapist via art mediums all lead to beneficial development. It helps youth with behavioral, emotional, and developmental issues by offering a creative, secure environment where they may start exploring their fears, anxieties, and emotions under the supervision and assistance of a licensed art therapist. It has a track record of successfully reaching even the most difficult teenagers!

What is the process of art therapy?

Creating art with a trained therapist at your side is art therapy. The art serves as a conduit for communication between the young person and the therapist, facilitating exchanges of ideas via spoken words or burgeoning artistic expression.

The artwork produced may also act as a transitional item, keeping the young person and therapist in communication both within and outside of sessions and offering a crucial degree of stability.

Art therapists are specially educated in psychotherapy as well as creative concepts, and they are aware of how creating art may help individuals express their emotions and ideas. They choose each creative arts project's supplies and theme in accordance with the unique requirements of each person. Building masks or puppets to talk about tough subjects, painting a portrait of how they believe others view them, building a collage about their thoughts, and sculpting or sketching an impression of what their fear, despair, or wrath looks like are a few examples.

Emotional Relief Through Music Therapy

Using music to assist people in achieving social and emotional objectives such as enhancing self-worth, lowering stress levels, controlling emotions, and raising self-awareness is known as music therapy. To achieve these objectives, teenagers may write lyrics for songs, perform music, play an instrument, listen to music, or create their own songs. Even while it may not seem important, producing songs, playing an instrument, or listening to music can be very soothing and have a big impact on a teen's path toward mental health.

Teens may benefit from music therapy in the following ways:

1. Enhancing one's perception of oneself

Teenagers sometimes let self-defeating beliefs control how they feel about themselves. They could believe that they are foolish, useless, or powerless, and these ideas may influence their behavior as well as their beliefs. They may fight these bad ideas by penning a song or picking up an instrument. Teens might realize they are valuable and have special skills and abilities by completing a difficult activity. They should be satisfied with themselves for taking on a task and succeeding even if they aren't the world's most skilled or great musicians.

2. Lowering Anxiety and Stress

It has been shown that making and listening to music may help people relax and feel less stressed. People with high anxiety levels may find it beneficial to listen to music. Teens may experience an increase in heart rate, shortening of breath, and a "fight or flight" reaction when they are worried. Teens may let go of tension by listening to and accepting the familiarity of their favorite song or by taking on a difficult piece of music on an instrument.

Emotional Relief Through Writing Therapy

Writing provides a multitude of avenues for expression. We may access our creative energy when we compose tales. We establish a secure area for emotional expression when we journal. Writing in a journal enables us to clarify and manage our emotions while also letting go of them. The more we write, the less we can worry. Reading past entries might also encourage introspection and help us understand the significance of the experiences that have impacted our lives. Some teenagers dislike journaling because they think someone else could discover it. Tell them it's OK to express their emotions in writing, then tear up the paper or erase the words from the computer. They may still arrange and let go of their emotions and ideas, thanks to it.

6.3 How to Step out of Comfort Zones for Growth

Our comfort zone is the place where we feel secure, at ease, unafraid, and satisfied. Things that are comfortable and familiar to us are found within our comfort zones. Furthermore, each of us has a unique comfort zone that lies outside of it. Consider all of the things you do without thinking about it, such as going on a stroll with a buddy or participating in a sport you like. These are activities that are simple and generally pleasant. While carrying on with such activities is OK, venturing outside of the comfort zone may result in a variety of rewarding and difficult experiences—that's where the development occurs! Which terms would you use to characterize situations that took you outside of your comfort zone? Moving from the known and comfortable to the strange and unexpected might make us feel uncomfortable, uncomfortable, scared, or even challenged. However, it may also be enjoyable, thrilling, and gratifying.

Recall your first day at SuperCamp, if you have gone, or your first day in a new school. Discovering your classroom, worried about your teacher's possible demeanor or whether they'll welcome you. Many of us are uncomfortable in certain situations and may be feeling a little stressed. However, what can be waiting for us beyond that comfort zone is a mentor, new buddy, or unforgettable educational opportunity. By stepping outside of our comfort zone, we may accomplish goals we might not have known we were passionate about!

List three things that you sometimes consider trying, but that would be outside of your comfort zone. Perhaps it's training for an athletic event, taking part in a play or concert, finishing a marathon, or climbing a mountain. Perhaps all it takes is putting up your hand in response to a question in class or making an introduction. Because it's familiar, simple, and, well, comfy, we may choose to remain in our comfort zones. Everything outdoors might seem dangerous and unpleasant. Remember,

- Little steps may lead to big ones. Every little step contributes to your comfort zone and makes it bigger in the long run.

- We must push our inner boundaries to discomfort to develop and thrive.

Furthermore, it's critical to keep in mind the role that image plays in this process. Fear of our image prevents us from being the people we want to be and from taking the actions that would improve our lives. This fear is known as self-image.

6.4 Mindful Practices for Teenagers

Being mindful extends beyond meditation. Any action, including walking, eating, and breathing, may be made more mindful by including this feeling of presence. Teenagers should practice mindfulness. You may stop, take a breath, and re-establish a connection with the world around you by practicing mindfulness. It might be the difference between a difficult and successful day to take a minute to check in with yourself and ground yourself, especially on days when life seems frantic. Follow the exercises listed below to enrich your day-to-day life.

- **Consume Healthy Food**

  Using all of our senses to thoroughly enjoy and savor our meal is the goal of mindful eating. We eat slowly, taking our time to appreciate the flavor, texture, aroma, and appearance of our food. Try incorporating mindful eating into at least one of your daily meals. Disconnect from outside distractions, set down your fork in between bites, and give every bite a true flavor.

- **Make deliberate movements.**

It is also possible to transform physical activity into a mindfulness practice. Whether you're stretching, doing tai chi, yoga, or other physical activities, mindful movement is being aware of your body's feelings as you move. Your muscles should contract and release when you feel your feet on the ground. When you become aware of every feeling while moving, it transforms into meditation.

- **Take conscious breaths.**

Exercises that focus on mindful breathing help us relax and improve our mental clarity by drawing our attention to the rhythm of our natural breath. Every day, try dedicating a short period to sit still and concentrate on your breathing. Pay attention to every breath in and out, feeling the rise and fall in your chest and abdomen. Gently return your thoughts to your breathing whenever they stray. You may become more focused and aware by doing breathing exercises for even one minute.

- **Consider practicing mindfulness while strolling.**

Walking meditation is a fantastic technique to stretch and move your body while also calming the mind since it blends mindfulness with physical exercise. Movement and mindfulness both enhance general well-being and relaxation.

Observe your body's movement, the rhythm of your breathing, and the feel of your feet hitting the earth as you stroll. You may practice walking meditation anyplace, even in your living room or a park.

- **Practice a body scan meditation class.**

  As a mindfulness activity, do a mental body scan, which examines your whole body from head to toe.

  Throughout your body, pay attention to any tight spots or uncomfortable spots. To encourage relaxation, consciously relax and soften such areas.

- **Give single-tasking priority.**

  Although multitasking has grown commonplace, it often lowers productivity and causes stress. Instead, consider single-tasking.

  Give each work your whole attention at a time. You'll probably discover that you're less anxious and more productive.

- **9. Write a list of thankfulness.**

  By encouraging us to concentrate on the good parts of our lives, this practice enables us to be happy and fulfilled.

  Make a thankfulness journal every day to record all the wonderful things, both large and small, in your life.

- **Engage in attentive hearing.**

  Relationships are strengthened, and communication is enhanced by mindful listening.

  The next time you're in a discussion, put all of your attention on the other person and ignore any outside distractions. Make sure you've thought out your response before answering.

Chapter 7

Support and Empowerment

Everyday existence might depress us and cause us to become sick of our situation. When our routines grow monotonous and uninteresting, we often find ourselves wondering where to find some freeing diversion. If you found your inner energy source, how would you respond? Daily workouts that build your endurance and strength might help you unleash your special power. In this chapter, you will learn all there is to know about support and empowerment.

7.1 Daily Practices for Self-empowerment

Daily workouts that build your endurance and strength might help you unleash your special power. You may access unexpected abilities inside yourself by engaging in these powerful practices:

Teenage self-care resources

- **Physical well-being is important.**

    Physical health is equally as important as mental health when it comes to self-care. Regular exercise has several advantages for young people, particularly if they spend most of their days inside. A 2015 meta-analysis found that teenagers' self-concept may be significantly impacted by physical exercise. A person's perception of their physical attractiveness—an area in which many teenagers struggle—is also tied to their self-concept. Engaging in regular physical exercise releases endorphins, which elevate mood in addition to increasing confidence. Our bodily systems are stressed out during exercise since it raises our heart rate. Thus, endorphins—which elevate our mood and lessen pain perception—are released into our body by our brain. In addition to supporting team sports and regular exercise, parents should assist teens in discovering new forms of movement. Regular physical exercise has been shown in studies to lessen the symptoms of stress, anxiety, depression, and other mental health issues.

- **Put your attention on self-compassion.**

Encourage your child to develop self-compassion rather than concentrating on their sense of self-worth. Self-compassion, or treating oneself with kindness, is a better alternative to self-esteem, claims researcher Kristen Neff. She discovered in her 2009 research that those who exhibited higher levels of self-compassion also reported feeling more content. The participants were pleasant to themselves, admitted their shortcomings, and embraced who they were.

How, therefore, may teens begin to develop more self-compassion? Encourage your adolescent to write down their positive attributes, even the little ones, for a few minutes each morning or evening. Whether it's a spa day, weekend getaway, or lunch meeting with a friend, giving your adolescent something to look forward to can help them feel more optimistic about the future. It might need more time and effort to practice self-compassion if your adolescent suffers from a mental health illness, such as significant depression or anxiety disorder. In case your child is experiencing emotions of despair or unworthiness, talk therapy may assist them in recognizing their positive traits and creating constructive coping mechanisms to counteract thoughts of negativity. Here are some more pointers to assist teens in developing compassion:

- **Encourage your child to express their emotions.**

  Everyone dealing with mental health issues should, particularly young people, raise awareness of their experiences without passing judgment. When your adolescent is sad, they may say something like, "I'm having a really hard time right now," to express how they feel. In this sense, people might begin to see their depression as a condition they are dealing with rather than a part of who they are.

- **Make use of positive affirmations.**

  Though they may seem like corny phrases best left on greeting cards, positive affirmations may be a simple but effective tool for reminding your adolescent of their value. Assist your teenager in selecting positive affirmations that are clear, grounded in reality, and, most importantly, sincere. Rather than saying, "Nothing will stop you," you may say something like, "There will be bad days as well as good ones, but you can always keep going." You may assist your teenager in developing more compassion by modeling self-compassion for them. Increased emotional resilience, less stress, and enhanced general well-being are all correlated with increased compassion. Helping your adolescent develop healthy habits may take some time, but emotional self-care may have a profound impact on their mental well-being.

- **Stay clear of societal comparisons.**

Setting objectives and maintaining motivation might sometimes be achieved by evaluating yourself against others. But no matter who we are or what we do, if we get fixated on the notion that the grass is always greener on the other side, we will always be the ones falling short. The comparison may have a detrimental effect on mental health, particularly for younger teenagers and adolescents who often perceive an "imaginary audience" and may feel as if everyone is watching them.

Sadly, comparisons might become unavoidable due to social networking sites. Studies have shown the connection between social media use and serious depressive disorders, anxiety disorders, and other mental health issues among teenagers. Furthermore, schools frequently serve to promote social comparison. The impediments and failures that are inevitable components of the learning process are not respected when students are tracked only on their academic achievement. Help your adolescent develop a fresh viewpoint so they can stop comparing themselves to other people. Ask them to consider a person they often use as a comparison for themselves. Next, reassure your adolescent that they are unable to live that person's life and that they have no evidence that the other person's life is superior. Encourage your child to limit their social media use and to limit or mute any accounts that they find especially upsetting when it comes to drawing unfavorable comparisons.

In the end, circumstances may not always mirror what is seen on the outside. Your adolescent will feel more secure in themselves and be able to avoid instinctively believing that they are inferior to others once they adjust their viewpoint to take this into account.

- **Assist your child in developing their strengths.**

  You can assist your adolescent in developing their strengths if you are aware of their abilities and capabilities. Susan Harter, a researcher, claims that teenagers' feeling of value is based on eight categories, such as social acceptability, romantic attractiveness, and athletic aptitude. This means that self-concept is domain-specific.

  Your daughter may believe she's not very athletic, but she seems to get excited about creative projects. Encouraging your teen to pursue options that align with their strengths helps foster a solid sense of self-worth. Fostering your teen's abilities might immediately improve their attitude in the short term. They get positive reinforcement for completing their task, which might take the form of verbal or material rewards. This enhances their feeling of self and fosters pride. Teenagers who excel in the subjects that are important to them experience a boost in self-worth and self-compassion. Teens may prevent the infiltration of negative ideas and self-worth concerns by focusing on their strengths.

- **Promote therapy as a self-care strategy.**

Although they're not always sufficient, encouraging healthy lifestyle modifications, getting enough sleep, taking up new interests, and engaging in other self-care activities may help your adolescent feel their best. If your adolescent is going through psychological difficulties, discuss with them the value of therapy as a kind of self-care.

Teens might be reluctant to talk about mental health issues, so it's important to be there for them at every stage of their journey, offering your undying love and support. Remind your child that experiencing occasional melancholy and worry are natural emotions. But it's important to get professional assistance if such emotions cause problems for them in their day-to-day lives. At any point in life, sticking to too much negativity may become draining. Not only that, but teens may find it more difficult to operate in daily life as a result of the symptoms of major depressive disorder, bipolar disorder, and other mental illnesses. Talk therapy is a helpful treatment for a variety of mental health issues and offers them a secure, encouraging setting in which to work through their emotions, create constructive coping mechanisms, and enhance their sense of self.

7.2 How to Celebrate Small Wins

Teens may greatly increase their self-esteem, maintain motivation, and build a positive outlook by acknowledging and appreciating their small victories. Teens might love these creative and fun methods to commemorate their small victories:

- **Make a Win Jar**

  Adorn a jar with a label that reads "Win Jar." Record your accomplishments on a little piece of paper and put them in the jar whenever you reach a goal. Take some time at the end of a month or a week to review your achievements and consider how far you've come.

- **Reward Yourself**

  When you reach a goal, treat yourself to a modest treat. It may be a particular treat, a go-to snack, or some downtime spent doing something you like.

- **Post on social media:**

  To let friends and family know about your accomplishments, publish them on social media. It's a means of getting compliments and support.

- **Give yourself a present as a surprise.**

Get yourself a fun surprise, such as a subscription box to your preferred clothes or cosmetics company, Winc Wine, or a blind date with a book—a wrapped book with just a few genre/plot hints on the wrapping.

- **Create a trophy for yourself.**

  Choose a trophy to symbolize your victory. With every next little (or major) victory, designate a new item as your trophy—it may be a succulent, a record, or a poster—and encourage yourself to do more.

7.3 How to Build a Support Network

A good support system is a network of individuals you can rely on, both practically and emotionally, and it goes beyond just having someone to weep on. A robust support system comprises medical personnel as well as a social network of individuals. Families and communities play a significant role in the human experience since we cannot thrive or live on our own. This is particularly true while facing difficulties and roadblocks in life, like parenting an adolescent undergoing therapy.

Adolescents with strong support networks benefit greatly from improved mental and physical health. For instance, they often experience feelings of sadness and anxiety less. This may be the case because those inside a support system pay attention and provide advice. You will probably feel less isolated and overwhelmed if you speak about your nervous emotions with close friends who are willing to listen. Your network of friends and family may be helpful to motivate you to obtain treatment for depression before it worsens.

Individuals who have strong social networks may also live longer and have fewer health issues. Having low levels of stress may help you retain better heart health since excessive levels of anxiety and stress can cause issues like high blood pressure. Furthermore, those with lower levels of stress may also be better able to maintain healthy routines, including frequent exercise, a balanced diet, and enough sleep.

Numerous additional advantages of having a strong support network include: • Improving your capacity for stress management.

- Diminish the harmful consequences of mental turmoil.

- Offer encouragement and optimism.

- Increase self-worth.

- Promote sensible decisions.

- Boost the likelihood of following a treatment plan.

You may only consider other teenagers to be part of your support network while you're a teen. A lot of teenagers indeed consider other teenagers to be their closest pals. But don't discount other individuals because of their status or age. You should think about adding the following individuals to your support network:

- Parents
- Siblings

- grandparents, aunts, uncles,

- coaches, pastors, volunteers at your place of worship, and neighbors.

You may include your pet in your network of support! Although they can't provide you with advice, your dog or cat can listen to your problems. What happens if you don't already have a network of friends and family that you could lean on for support? To meet the right kind of people for you, you may need to give some of the activities you may participate in some thought. You may meet upbeat, encouraging individuals at volunteer work, in an after-school program, or via part-time employment.

How To Build Up Your Support System

After selecting a few individuals to be part of your support network, you should start learning how to assist them when they need it and how to depend on them in times of need. Be patient with yourself; asking for assistance might be tough. Starting with sharing life's blessings with your selected support system could be an excellent idea. Tell folks, for instance, if you ace a test in a class, you've been having trouble with. Inform others that you are in treatment for drug addiction after you have been clean for thirty days, three months, or a year.

People will open up to you when you take down your guard and become more vulnerable with them. Just two or one person in your support network should come to mind as someone you are at ease confiding in. Take a deep breath and ask for assistance from those folks if you are struggling to digest anything in your life or if you just need some advice on what to do next. They'll probably feel privileged that you think highly enough of them to confide in them.

How To Manage And Foster Your Support System

Being a helpful buddy is crucial if you want to keep your support network intact over time. Give the individuals in your life who matter a lot of time. This includes answering calls and sending SMS back. Say hello if you haven't heard from them in a long time. Be available for someone in the support group who needs someone to listen to them or ask you for a little favor. The saying "You can only have a buddy by being a friend" may be familiar to you. This is especially true when it comes to the network of support; if you don't stick by them while they're struggling, they won't want to help you get through it. Some individuals may inevitably go, and others will join your support network as you grow. Try not to take things too personally; everyone experiences this at some point in their lives due to the universal rhythm of life. Just make sure you have someone you can always rely on to assist you through the many challenges life throws at you and to hold you up.

7.4 Embracing Your Paths to Growth

Accepting change is a vital component of human development. We may use the power of change to our advantage by using it as a catalyst for resilience, flexibility, and self-improvement rather than fighting it out of fear or uncertainty. In the quest for personal development, change is not the adversary; rather, it is our friend. Keep in mind that every transition life throws at you gives you a different chance for personal growth and development. If you approach change with a willingness to learn and a growth attitude, you'll discover that you're on a meaningful and gratifying road of personal progress.

There was a time when you used to have those large, gorgeous eyes and those little hands with short fingers. You recall another occasion when you were unable to walk or crawl, and you turned over and fell out of the chair. You were crying so much because of the agony, and your mother had to hug you. Allow me to relive the moments when your parents enrolled you in elementary school for the first time. You were wearing shorts or this huge dress. You were always in tears because you didn't want your mother to abandon you to those weird-looking instructors. You must also have remembered all the insane things you unintentionally did when you were between the ages of six and seven.

Entering your adolescence, you're happy to be called a teenager. Teens should feel free to be joyful, joyful, and joyful, but there are several things you should avoid doing at that point in your life. The adolescent years span from 13 to 19 years of age. Over the years, you face a lot of challenges, disappointments, joys, and hardships; the objective is to be able to overcome them all. Being an early teenager—that is, being between the ages of 13 and 15—means that you should be aware that your outlook on life and how you respond to problems should vary from that of a person who is ten years old. You should stop being such a baby and work on changing your thinking. You can't automatically start jumping ships and exposing your heart just because you're a teenager. Remain composed and mindful of your surroundings.

As I said before, adolescence is an exciting and joyful time, but you should use caution while enjoying yourself. A genuine buddy is not someone who just grins and jokes around with you. You should choose carefully whom you will spend your adolescent years with as a young teen. Those who share your objective. Individuals who would be thrilled to see you succeed. As you approach adolescence, you could begin to think things like, "Oh, I'm a teenager now, I can party with friends," "I can have a boyfriend," "I can go wherever I want without telling my parents, "And anything else that comes to mind. These aren't horrible ideas, but right now, that's not what counts.

You must consider how to be the finest version of yourself. Ways to be ready for what is ahead. It's never too early to start planning for the future, I promise. It makes your life simple and organized and offers you an advantage over others. To have the best adolescent years possible, you must have the proper mentoring and direction. You have now entered the late teens and have had a taste of adolescence. You are used to the feelings, and all that adolescence has to offer. It will take you a few years to reach adulthood. What plans do you have for when you grow up?

Age is a lie! You're kidding if you believe you still have a long life ahead of you and that you are still young! Nobody is too young to start saving for the future. This is where you start! You should act like an adult as a late adolescent, make important decisions, and consider options carefully. Have the courage to take personal responsibility. Do you still believe that your parents will take care of everything? That is a jest! From this day forward, even if you are not yet an adult, you must assume responsibilities. Don't let your past hinder your potential to succeed. My coach has always said that it is not your fault if you were raised in a low-income household or if you were born into one, but it will be your responsibility if you live out your senior years there. Act now! You should be cautious about who you roll with as a late teen. The individuals you choose to remain in your firm with. People that place an equal value on things are what you need. People who share your goal of reaching the same objective. These will enable you to make the proper decisions and develop into the finest version of yourself. Steer clear of pointless rivalry among your classmates. Whoa! My acquaintance is well-known, wealthy, and the recipient of several endorsements. I have to emulate her and surpass her. These are all pointless competitions that might divert your attention from your objective and force you to pursue unsuitable endeavors. It's OK to want to be like someone you look up to. However! Do not let the desire to emulate someone else consume you as you attempt to become that person. Remain loyal to your identity! Take full advantage of your adolescent years and embrace them but remember to act responsibly and maturely.

Chapter 8

Parents and Educators Guide

Teens and their parents or teachers may find it difficult to deal with adulthood. Significant social, emotional, and physical growth is occurring at this period. You will discover what a parent or instructor can do to support a teen's well-being in this chapter.

8.1 Understanding The Teenage Brain

Preteens and adolescents have moods or feelings of ups and downs, much as adults do. Preteens and young people, for instance, may experience ups and downs as well as happy moments. Additionally, they often want more alone time or seclusion. These emotional ups and downs might occur more often and with greater intensity throughout the preteen and adolescent years. The emotional ups and downs that your kid experiences might be caused by a variety of factors, including psychological, emotional, social, and physical ones. It's common for neither you nor your kid to be able to pinpoint the exact reason for their mood swings. Moods are an indication that your kid is striving to comprehend and regulate increasingly complicated adult emotions. This is a crucial stage in the development of teenagers. To support your kid through this stage of their adult journey, you have a significant role to play.

Why do Emotional ups and downs happen?

Many factors are involved in the regulation of emotions a teen faces. Some of them are listed below:

- **Physical factors**

  Adolescence is a time of many bodily changes for preteens and adolescents. Your kid may feel self-conscious or uncomfortable about the changes to their body, or they may just desire more solitude and alone time. Teenagers and preteens who seem to be maturing more quickly or slower than their peers may have emotional responses to these physical changes.

  Sleep is another bodily component. Teenagers need 8 to 10 hours of sleep, whereas preteens require 9 to 11 hours. Your child's mood is probably going to be impacted by how much sleep they receive. Moods may also be influenced by your child's food habits, nutritional status, and degree of physical exercise. Eating well and getting plenty of exercise may frequently help your kid learn to control their emotions.

- **Brain factors**

  During adolescence, the adolescent brain undergoes several changes. For instance, your child's body produces sex hormones as a result of brain abnormalities. These hormones cause emotions of passion and lust as well as physical changes. For your youngster, these novel emotions may be strong and perhaps perplexing.

  Furthermore, your child's brain will continue to develop until their early 20s. The prefrontal cortex, the final region of the brain to mature, is intimately linked to the parts of the brain in charge of controlling and handling emotions. This implies that your youngster may become more emotionally reactive than usual and may struggle to control some of their stronger emotions. They're still getting used to processing and expressing their feelings in mature ways.

- **Social and emotional factors**

How your kid feels may be influenced by new ideas, feelings, friends, and obligations. As your child gets closer to independence, they are learning how to handle more challenges on their own. In addition, your child is spending more time focusing on themselves and their problems, such as school, friendships, and family dynamics. Stressful circumstances in the home might also impact your child's mood.

Assisting preteens and adolescents to experience more highs than lows

There are a few things you can do to encourage your kid to experience more highs than lows. Identifying the things your kid already appreciates is the first step. These might include engaging in their preferred sport, hanging out with long-time friends, listening to or performing music, sketching, making original digital material, and so on. Maintaining these routines will provide your youngster with a sense of security and a foundation for pursuing new interests. Additionally, you may assist your kid in discovering new pursuits that will test them, encourage goal-setting, and introduce them to new people.

These may include taking up a new hobby or joining a social club. Instead of assigning your kid these tasks, you may acquire ideas from hearing what they have to say about their likes and dislikes.

Assisting adolescents and preteens in coping with emotional ups and downs

Your youngster will always feel depressed or flat. However, parents have a lot of options for supporting their kids in adjusting to life's ups and downs.

- **Adopting a kid who can tolerate ups and downs**

Understanding that emotional ups and downs are a natural part of life might benefit your kid. Disclosing to your youngster that you feel flat too on sometimes is one of the finest methods to do this. It's also critical that your kid understands that they can turn to you in difficult situations or when they're feeling down. You are not required to resolve your child's issues. Saying something like, "I see you're having a difficult day," might be helpful instead. This teaches your youngster that it's OK to feel depressed or hopeless sometimes.

- **Maintaining contact with your kid**

It will be easier for you to identify the reasons behind your child's emotional ups and downs if you stay in touch and pay attention to what's happening in their lives. The finest moments for your kid to share things with you might sometimes be found during informal, daily activities like watching TV together or taking them somewhere.

- **Providing your kids with space**

  Your child is growing up, becoming independent, and trying new things. Try to give your child some space or time alone during this period so they may reflect on their newfound feelings and experiences. Inform your youngster that you are there for them to speak to.

- **Delaying the implementation of solutions**

  If there is an issue, talking with your kid about solutions might be beneficial, but they must feel like they "own" the answers and be involved in them. If your kid believes they are the source of the answer, they are also more inclined to attempt it. In addition, problem-solving is an important life skill that your kid will improve with practice. Fostering your child's ability to solve problems shows them that you appreciate their opinion while making choices that will impact their life.

8.2 How to Support Your Teens

- **Encourage acceptance of oneself.**

  Parents may play a significant role in fostering high self-esteem and self-acceptance in their children by encouraging them to pursue hobbies and abilities, emphasizing the need to establish reasonable goals, and creating effective strategies to reach them. Parents can assist children in developing a good self-image that will enable them to overcome obstacles more skillfully.

- **Talk about uncomfortable feelings.**

Recognize the norms of society and provide them the tools they need to deal with challenging emotions when they arise. Encourage your kid to express their emotions in constructive ways, like writing, music, or painting, by having a conversation with them about their feelings. Seek methods to stay in touch with your teenager. You may say something like "I understand," "That makes sense," or "It sounds like a difficult situation" in response to them opening up to you. Assure them that you are always available to them and that you are interested in learning about their thoughts and feelings. We learn to be mindful of our mental and emotional states by being aware of and paying attention to the tiny things in life. Positive well-being is also proven to be promoted by sharing our gratitude. We parents can express our gratitude.

- **Build Relationships.**

Studies indicate that positive family dynamics may lower an adolescent's risk of mental health problems. Mental wellness depends on us making time for the people who matter most in our lives and maintaining healthy relationships with family, friends, peers, and coworkers. Your youngster should be encouraged to form new acquaintances and stay in touch with their existing pals. This relationship aids their feeling of belonging. Encourage them to join a sports team, volunteer, be an active part of the school community, or simply spend time with their families to help them develop meaningful connections with others. It's also essential to know how to handle disagreements in partnerships.

- **Encourage the development of healthy coping mechanisms for stress and anxiety.**

If your adolescent is becoming irritated, discuss solutions together. Find out from your kid how they plan to handle disagreement on their own. They must also realize that everyone experiences stress from time to time and that certain stress is healthy stress that enhances performance. Putting things in perspective may also be achieved by discussing the worst-case scenario.

- **Set screen time limits.**

The new standard is interacting online via social networking sites, gaming apps, and texting. When you combine this with greater exposure to violence, incorrect body images, and online bullying, it becomes easy to see why it is so difficult for today's youth to develop and maintain healthy mental health. Overuse of screens promotes inactivity, wastes time that might be used to relieve exam stress, hinders the development of in-person connections, and, most crucially, results in inadequate sleep. Although it is one of the most difficult tasks for parents, it may also have the greatest effect on mental health.

- **Steer clear of power battles.**

  Teens may be finding it difficult to maintain control at the moment since the world seems so uncertain. As challenging as it may be at the time, try to understand their need to take charge instead of trying to suppress their ideas. Never bring up a topic when you're upset. Take a deep breath and walk away. You can speak to your kid about it later, and when you are both calm, the discussion will be far more fruitful. This demonstrates to your adolescent how you handle your feelings.

8.3 How to Create a Safe Emotional Environment

Many families find the adolescent years to be challenging. Young individuals can acquire opinions, values, and beliefs that diverge from their parents. This is a typical step in the process of becoming self-sufficient. Depending on the age and situation, parents may find it difficult to determine how much independence is appropriate for their kids. This is not treatable with medication. Since every young person is unique, they need distinct guidance. Contrary to speaking with younger children, communicating with teens may lead to conflict and tension. The teenager and you may have better communication if you adhere to a few easy recommendations.

Maintaining open channels of communication is crucial. Among the recommendations are:

- Pay more attention than you talk; keep in mind that every one of us has one mouth and two ears. This serves as a reminder that listening should take up twice as much time as talking. This is particularly crucial when speaking with teens, who could open up to us more if we wait to speak for a while.

- Set aside time to spend together. Although teens are often preoccupied with school, friends, and other activities, you may still talk to them during supper and breakfast. Offer to drive them somewhere or pick them up from somewhere; this will open up more conversational avenues.

- Allow them some privacy; teens need their area. For instance, knock before entering their room.

- Stay up to date with their hobbies by attending their sporting practice sessions, watching television programs with them, and listening to their music. Maintain your involvement in their lives.

- Be a kind parent and educator: Adolescence is a period when adolescents often struggle with their evolving sense of self and need affection. Inform them often. Use whatever physical touch they feel comfortable with to express your affection. Honor their accomplishments, provide forgiveness for their errors, pay attention to their problem-solving strategies, and express interest in finding a solution. Encourage them to solve problems. All young people need to feel unique and included to have a strong sense of self-worth.

- Have fun and schedule downtime for relaxation and jokes. Positive emotions facilitate effective communication.

8.4 How to Working Together for the Emotional Health of a Teenager

A well-rounded kid has to be raised with a great deal of patience, openness to learning, and active involvement from all of the important adults in the child's life. For the efforts of these stakeholders—parents and teachers—to be successful, they must collaborate well. Establishing a healthy parent-teacher connection seems to be hampered most by a lack of communication. It seems that in a parent-teacher connection, neither party listens to the other, which has a detrimental effect on the child's development.

- The first step in closing this gap is to adopt a new viewpoint. You must begin to see your opponent as a friend rather than a danger. It is advisable to follow a teacher's guidance at home and to take a parent's counsel into account while interacting with the child at school.

- Recognizing that neither the instructor nor the parent is privy to the whole narrative is crucial. Thus, the knowledge that the parents and the instructor have is complimentary, and together, they bring the story to a close.

- A shift in viewpoint must be supported by action. Parent-teacher conferences should be held in person or regularly to promote active communication. The specifics of the student's emotional and intellectual development at home and school should be discussed in these sessions.

- School systems can arrange parent-teacher conferences that include a predetermined agenda and a free-flowing discussion at the conclusion. This increases parent involvement and gives educators and parents a chance to strengthen their communities.

- Role-playing days are an innovative way to introduce parents to the challenges of teaching. These days, parents assume the role of educators and recognize the difficulties involved in overseeing a whole class.

The modern parenting team now includes the instructor, the mother, and the father. Accept this reality and work together to create the ideal environment for developing intellectual ability.

Conclusion

The years of teenage years, which last from 12 to 24 years of age, are an incredible time of development. Teenagers have a variety of novel emotional situations that test their capacity to manage a wide range of strong emotions. Young kids need to learn how to deal with emotionally charged circumstances that might be unpleasant without harming themselves or other people. Emotional maturity is intimately linked to self-awareness and values awareness. During adolescence, this self-identity evolves and becomes more definite. When teenage children grow from infancy into maturity, they undergo enormous changes in every area of their lives. Socially, teenagers' main source of support moves from their family to their friends as their demand for independence grows. Youth are particularly vulnerable to peer pressure because of the growing significance of peer interactions (meaning to adhere to the norms of the peer group). This book's main goal was to teach teenagers how they can explore and transform their inner world through various practices. This book also teaches the parents and other carers the fundamental knowledge they need to understand and accept teenagers' natural developmental growth. Equipped with this knowledge, parents and other educators will also feel more effective and confident as they help their kids navigate these often challenging and perplexing years.

www.ingramcontent.com/pod-product-compliance
Lightning Source LLC
Chambersburg PA
CBHW071223260726
48653CB00042B/1809